# Hood Medical:
# This Is Why I Sing

Barbara J. Barre

'Hood Medical: This Is Why I Sing

© 2019 Barbara J Barrett,
BeyondCategory Publishing
Cleveland, Ohio USA 2019

Please see your healthcare practitioner in a timely
manner for any personal health issues.

Cover design Kareem Barrett & Barbara Barrett

Artwork Malcolm Barrett & Bakari Lyles

Photographs by Barbara J. Barrett

ISBN-13: 978-1-7332606-0-2

# DEDICATION

'Hood Medical is dedicated to regular people. Sometimes life and situations are deep, sometimes not. But always, it is what it is, and wherever you go, there you are. When we accept these givens as far as humankind, we will have taken the first steps towards acceptance, adjustments, healing and making this a better world to live in.

# CONTENTS

# BEGIN WITH GRATITUDE

First, thanks be to God and the Heavenly Hosts for faith, hope, persistence and stamina. Many thanks and gratitude to my sister, Patricia Lyles, and my brother, Theodore J Burns III for their encouragement and enthusiasm with this project. Thanks to my mother Donnie M. Burns, affectionately known as Agent 93, for her support and proofreading, and for always insisting on correct spelling and grammar from me through the years. Except now. In some parts of this document. (You'll understand when you get to What's That Mean, Tho?) Continuing with gratitude, thanks to my dad Theodore J. Burns Jr, rest his soul, who persevered with his projects until he could not. He was a great example! My cousin, Helen Carmona Palmer, persistently encouraged me to write this book and helped with the editing. I appreciate your confidence in me! Thanks also to my cousin Linda Callaway RN, for giving me a very appropriate and personal strategy of sorts, for becoming a registered nurse. A special thank you to my sons, Kareem and Malcolm, who unknowingly persevered with me through the earliest parts of my nursing career and through my pitfalls. I love and appreciate you very much.

In keeping with the diverse nature of a large metropolitan area, I saw and attended to all different races and ethnicities of patients, students and families. This was made easier because my personal experiences with other races while growing up were not traumatizing or threatening. There were no feelings of inferiority implied, inferred or taught in my family. Aside from sometimes wishing to be offered opportunities that some others were offered, I never wanted to be anyone or anything other than who I was. For this, I again thank my parents, grandparent, other extended family members and my ancestral lineage.

Thanks to my hospital, homecare, "out in the field" patients and school chilrens (yes, I said chilrens, that's not a typo) for keeping it real at all times. Thanks to the variety of wonderful staff and supervisors I worked with over the years. Thank you to the many parents who do their best on a daily basis, despite obstacles, to raise their children into competent and confident adults. Your children provide hope for our future. Thank you also to the adults who are committed to maintaining their own optimal health.

Finally, I'd like to express a large chunk of gratitude to Dr. E. Louis Priem who was the head doctor over the SICU at the no longer existent Mt. Sinai Medical Center in the heart of one of Cleveland's best known 'hoods. He was committed to having nurses and other staff on board who looked like members of the surrounding community. He gave us chances, knowing and expecting that all of us could and would be, fully and equally competent. He was an exemplary leader and I'm extremely grateful to have worked under his guidance, particularly during one of my pitfalls which you'll read about later.

# I DIDN'T DO IT! (DISCLAIMER)

Seriously, I have no reason to make these stories up, and I have not. As you'll see, I can recount a funny story, but some of these are not the least bit funny. Some stories are relatively recent, while some happened twenty-five years ago, or more. To ensure privacy, I may have changed the gender and or other specifics to protect the innocent, the goofy, the aging (myself included) and the otherwise helpless or innocent, in these matters of stress, illness and sometimes humor.

I am a registered nurse, not a doctor. There's a big licensing difference, even though I've learned a lot and even though when working in nursing, it's not uncommon for some people to want to treat me like a doctor.

*Please, if you have **any** questions on a medical issue, consult with your licensed healthcare professional in a timely manner. This book is **not** meant to diagnose or prescribe a treatment.*

# 'HOOD GLOSSARY (WHATS THAT MEAN, THO??)

OK. I know some of you are going to think parts of this book are written with some of the worst language and grammar, ever. Well, 'Hood Medical: This is Why I Sing is partially written in what I call inner-city, 'hood, African American vernacular, otherwise known as Ebonics. Some stories would lose their flavor if they were written in 100% correct and proper English, spelling, grammar and sentence structure. Besides, I was using Ebonics long before it was coined as such.

Please be clear when I say, my mother, Agent 93 would be sure to correct me when she heard it. I got excellent grades in English and spelling, and I knew what was correct and incorrect. It's just that even back then, pre-Ebonics felt so comfortable and was so much fun!

The definitions of slang, colloquialisms, vernacular, neologism, even Jamaican patois, all imply using a more common, relaxed, informal, locally understood and used language. With that in mind, let's go over some of the terms you may hear as you "listen in text" to some of the conversations I'll share! This is your mini-glossary and it'll be fun! (Don't be side eyeing me. I can already see some of y'alls faces turning up.) Here we go...

- bruh = brother, oftentimes used amongst men who

know each other well

- wayment = wait a minute
- talmbout = talking about
- finna = fixing to, as in getting ready to
- imabouta = also means I'm getting ready to
- dope = the epitome of cool, awesome, that's what's up
- doing the most = go sit'choself down somewhere cuz you doing too much
- extra = same as above
- sit'choself = sit yourself, as in sit down (they really say, "sit'choass" down)
- issa = it's a ("issabouta" = it's about to...)
- ight = alright. Think of "alright" and say it minus the A, the L and the R
- turnt = having a ridiculous amount of fun. Also "turnt up" or "turn up"

Not to worry though, I did not use all of those, often. That would have been too much, and the spell check thingy was already losing its cyber mind. But I did choose stories that allowed me to most effectively speak in the patient, client, or student's voice. My hope is, this way, you get optimal feel for the scenario.

Above all, please remember Ebonics is a language all to itself. Its usage does not imply ignorance. To me it's a form of being bilingual and in my case, it helps with my ability to relate in certain circumstances. All African Americans do not choose Ebonics, but this is part of African American culture. Just as when we go to France, we can speak French, or go to Nigeria with the Yoruba people, we may speak Yoruba, we can still speak and write what's considered correct and proper English and use Ebonics. If you wanna... sorry. If you want to read some funny stuff, hashtag Ebonics on Instagram! #ebonics

# 1 WHAT HAD HAPPENED FIRST WAS...

"There is no greater agony than bearing an untold story inside you." –Maya Angelou

Someone asked me why I wanted to call my memoir 'Hood Medical. The reference to living in the hood is frequently assumed to mean the inner city, or even a ghetto. The term hood can have a negative connotation. But any community located within a large city or metropolitan area, can be referred to as a hood, short for neighborhood.

As I look back on my thirty-plus year nursing career, I notice a good portion of my nursing work took place in larger, inner-city teaching hospitals; by way of inner-city home healthcare visits and in our urban metropolitan school district. They are some of the best places to work if you like adventure, variety, the unusual and have a desire to continue learning as you're working. You also get to work with a variety of people, all genders, races, ethnicities, and ages. Even with regard to specializing in a specific medical area, the chances for learning are huge. As you'll see, I "specialized" for a few years in a couple of departments, but fulfillment for me came through variety.

Neighborhoods can have as much diversity, color and character, as the people who live in them. Across the city of Cleveland, there is much diversity. The Cuyahoga River had been credited or faulted, whichever you want to say, with ethnically and racially dividing Cleveland proper. This has changed significantly over the years. While I was growing up and attending school, I experienced having one or two white students in my upper elementary through high school classes. This was a huge change from when my family moved into our house. I got to witness white flight first-hand, even though at age five, I did not understand why.

It was all good however, because families in our neighborhood were working professionals, with some stay at home moms. The neighborhood was orderly, and the adults were in charge. The streetlights were the indicators that it was time to come in, and we respected adults, lest there be repercussions. Stay at home moms like my mother, were very aware of activities going on during the day; fathers were informed of any misbehavior after mothers dished out their share of discipline; and there were further repercussions because dads did not take any mess, either. When support was needed, it most often was received. The homes were well kept, and as children, we were for the most part, happy and not fearful.

Then came my college days, and I settled in nicely at the University of Cincinnati's College Conservatory of Music. I pledged Delta Sigma Theta, one of the largest African American sororities, and began to overcome my shyness. All was well until I began my student teaching in vocal music. With the onset of that experience came the sound of screeching tires coming to a swift halt in my brain. I did NOT want to teach music. I honestly never did. I really wanted to perform. However, due to the times and experiences of my parents and others in positions of guidance, I selected a program of education. Student teaching was so not it! "I think I'll go to plan B and apply to the nursing school right across the street from campus" I thought to myself. I did and got accepted. I figured I'd come up with a plan for music later, and this time it would be performing.

But all of that was shot down when I informed my parents of my last-minute desire to change, and they told me to come home after commencement because I didn't know what I was doing. They were right. I had no plan of action except that I did not want to teach in anyone's classroom as a way of making my living. I graduated with my bachelor's in education but did not do the classroom for several reasons. Aside from always wanting to perform, I was not ready to teach. I tended towards being shy, naïve, and insecure. Despite my personality challenges, I still was the product of a family that had expectations and discipline. I was not prepared for permissiveness in the behaviors of many school children, some of whom were only four years younger than me. It was more than I wanted to deal with.

Upon returning to Cleveland after graduation, I joined the Cleveland Orchestra and Blossom Festival Choruses, got married, had my first son, and went to a wonderful hospital school of nursing near downtown Cleveland. My cousin mentioned earlier, Linda Carmona Calloway, BSN, RN, suggested a hospital school as opposed to another baccalaureate program. It was a great suggestion for me because there was a nursing shortage and there were financial perks to help us get through. Hospital schools provided more clinical nursing and were great for someone who had no medical experience. I remained there after graduation for the first two years of my nursing practice.

On an affectionate, amusing note, I remember Linda telling me how her elderly Aunt used to call the hospital asking the operator for Nurse Carmona when she used to work nights. We used to laugh out loud about that because she said no one would call looking for Nurse anybody! But the hospital operators got to know who Aunt Jessie was, and would put her through. I thought about this story when deciding how to brand myself, thus Nurse Barbara, or #nursebarbara

After my first two years of practice at my alma mater, and about a year in neurology/neurosurgery, I settled into my favorite Surgical Intensive Care Unit at the old Mt Sinai Medical Center, while filling in as a PRN (Pro re nata, or as needed nurse) around the county. After a bit, the needs of my family took precedence, and I left the 12-hour shifts and started working for the Cleveland Metropolitan School District (CMSD). It was because of my degree in education that I was hired as a school nurse. Cousin Linda's strategy was good!

Nursing has been a wonderful, remarkable experience. My most profound memories came from hospital nursing; some of the strangest came through working out in the community (home care, EAP, cruising); but by far, most of my fondest memories come from public school nursing in metropolitan Cleveland and surrounding communities. Working with children for over 25 years has opened my eyes to the plight of families across racial and ethnic lines. The migration of families back and forth across Cleveland's Cuyahoga River has softened what once were pretty hard lines of racial division. The children, affectionately referred to as my "lil chilrens" belonged to me, too. Nursing with children had the most impact on me because I viewed myself as a second mom during school hours.

When I consider thirty plus years of nursing practice, I realize just how many people have come into my life, and how we left an impact on each other. From the funny stories to the tragic ones, my experiences helped me grow and mature, and realize just how blessed I am even through difficulties. The experiences and difficulties I'll be sharing, whether they were mine or those of my patients, have made me stronger. While learning to endure my own difficulties has certainly been a necessary thing, helping others through theirs has allowed me to see things from a perspective of an outsider. This means, a less emotional but still concerned approach. When you're on the other side of the fence looking in, particularly as a care provider, your vision can be clearer and not caught up in the emotions.

As far arts and creativity? They are the underlying forces that drive and sustain me, especially solo vocal performance. The arts are what have allowed me to remain positive in the face of so much of the negativity that illness and disease can bring. Singing helps me heal and minister through sound, lyrics, vibration, and passion. Dance is passion through movement. Dance and singing help me maintain a good caregiver relationship with my patients, students and clients, and help me stay grounded.

Here's to healing arts! May there always be a partnership between art and healing. This is why I sing.

## 2 IN THE HOSPITAL

### An Apple a Day

My white dress and nursing cap were fresh and sparkling. So was my disposition as a new nurse. I was well trained, although a bit concerned. "What if I don't know enough" I asked one of my nursing professors? "As long as you keep that attitude and stay on top of your learning, you'll do just fine," she answered.

Mr. Williams was 92 years old and had never had a hospital admission. And for his first time, I don't remember what treatment we gave him aside from some oxygen via nasal cannula, which is a plastic tubing used to allow oxygen to flow from a wall or tank source to the patient. He was pretty stable.

His wife was 15 or 20 years younger than he. She and I engaged in pleasant conversations during his stay. For some reason, one day we started talking about meal preparation for our families. "He worked in the West Virginia coal mines for almost 50 years" she said. "Every day he wanted a lard sandwich on white bread, a thermos of black coffee, and an apple for lunch. The trick is, you have to slice the lard while it's cold."

I don't know if my mouth dropped open, if it was twisted in horror at the thought of a lard sandwich, or what. But in my new nurse mind, gunshots went off as the whole concept of high cholesterol levels, and grease being horrible for you, were shot down. This man looked 15 or more years younger than his 90-something-year-old self and he had maintained it in part with a saturated animal fat sandwich, at least five days a week for years. Fat obtained from the adipose tissue of pigs. The dreaded swine. On white bread no less. I remember Wonder bread being so soft and pliable that as children, we would make bread balls out of it by smooshing it up with our fingers. But, that pork though; I still love bacon to this day.

And add to that, about a half quart of caffeine. Remember those thermoses that were about a foot tall? Yeah those. No herb tea, decaf coffee, nut milk, water or juice in there. Straight up caffeine!

But alas, those apples made it all better. I guess an apple a day really does keep the doctor away at least until you're 90. Even after eating so much of the dreaded swine.

## Smoking, Drinking, You're Not Thinking

I've been trying to figure out why smoking was ever allowed on hospital floors. Clearly that's proof I graduated from nursing school back in the olden days.

We had this one patient who was a regular admission. To this day, I even remember his name. Dude would come in and be on oxygen by nasal cannula or mask, coming from a wall source. However, he would disconnect the oxygen and wheel his IV (intravenous) out into the hallway on a pole so he could smoke his cigarette. And we'd let him, even if we didn't want to, because it was not against hospital policy, and it was within his rights, even if it made no sense.

Would you like to know his diagnosis? Emphysema. One of the chronic obstructive pulmonary diseases, or COPD. I know there are other factors besides smoking that contribute to emphysema and other lung issues. Chemical pollutants for example, can be contributors. But it's been proven and documented that smoking is a huge factor in its development and smoking contributes in a major way to the patient's demise.

I still find it hard to believe that we had to have a policy to enforce no smoking in a hospital. Especially since secondary smoke potentially affected all the other patients on the floor. Continuous exposure to even secondary smoke is said to increase the risk of heart disease. He was not the only smoker, but I remember him because of his diagnosis of lung disease. I guess the good part is, at least he didn't blow himself up. That's why he had to have the oxygen unhooked and the IV made portable. Oxygen, sparks, and flames do not mix well!

On a similar note, I once made a home visit where a different patient was on oxygen and smoked. The day I visited, the oxygen company rep came and changed the oxygen tank. The patient had just gotten out of the hospital and was being compliant by wearing his nasal cannula. But why, oh why, did he suddenly take the cannula, and suppress it under his chin, saying "Sorry Miss, I gotta have me a smoke." WTH (what the heck) I was thinking to myself as I hurried up and had him sign off on his paperwork and high tailed it out of his apartment! Clearly, by the way he had figured out how to suppress the oxygen, this was not the first time he had done this while technically hooked up to the tank. And I'm sure some reading this will think to themselves "there's not that much oxygen flowing through that tubing, and that flame from the lighter isn't that intense, so it can't start a fire." WHATEVER.

Then there was the lady who would repeatedly try to get me to bring her cigarettes when I'd come for her home visit. Who, me? Your nurse who does not smoke, and you have a lung issue? I'll bring you some bacon, but cigarettes?

No. JUST NO.

## Iced Pee

At one point, I was working on a neurology/neurosurgery floor that included admissions for alcoholics in delirium tremens (DTs). There was a pattern involved in this whole process. Toward the end of the month when funds get low, it meant there was no money to get that drink on, which resulted in withdrawal symptoms. We would see the same people repeatedly.

The interesting thing was, we had nurse/patient relationships with them, but the substance would sometimes cause them to turn on us. In the case of alcoholic beverages, they are called spirits for a reason. Threatening us while walking down the hallway half or fully naked, being loud and belligerent and needing sometimes to be in soft or even leather restraints, were commonplace occurrences. So was occasionally taking them into a corner in their room while we verbally reminded them of where they were and that we weren't having any foolishness. They got it; we understood each other. They were not usually crazy, just amped up because they were missing their chemical fix.

One day I think I saved a patient from an awful experience. It would have been his fault, but still. He was not in his right mind. As I got ready to tidy up his bed while he was out of the room, I noticed his water and ice pitcher on the floor under the bed. "Where did he get iced tea from?" I thought to myself. As I picked the pitcher up, I got an awful feeling. A closer look and sniff confirmed it. Yes, there was ice floating in it because oftentimes, we would fill the pitcher with ice and let it melt down so it would be cold. But this wasn't iced tea. Try iced pee. Sorry. I mean, urine. And yes, dark because remember, this was a long time alcoholic. Dude had peed in his water pitcher instead of getting up going to the bathroom, which was right next to his bed.

The thought of the patient drinking out of that pitcher, shot my very low to non-existent vomit reflexes through the roof. Yes, he was one who would from time to time threaten to kick our butts, but we knew him, were not afraid of him, and we knew why he acted the way he did. By the time the DTs had run their course, he was calm, sensible, withdrawn, almost embarrassed and even borderline remorseful. That experience made me feel really bad for him. What if I hadn't caught it and he tasted it? And what else was he doing that was kind of insane, when he was not in the hospital?

Research points to persistent substance abuse as being a serious problem with decision making.

## A Mother's Last Words

On the same floor, we had a specialized, enclosed, four-bed unit for more critical patients. Admitted to that area were men and women who had recently suffered a stroke, or who had a spinal cord injury. The interesting thing about strokes is you never really know the extent of the residual or lasting effect the stroke is going to have on the patient.

A lady in her forties or fifties was admitted for a stroke. Her daughters came to visit her and of course were very distraught, particularly since their mother could not talk. Well, most of the time she couldn't. Or just didn't.

At the time of her admission, I was on the day shift. For whatever reason, when I would go in to greet her at 6:50 in the morning, she would answer me and say good morning. Never opened her eyes to look at me, but she would speak clearly.

Although there seems to be no scientific data to prove it, in nursing school, we were always told, despite a patient's condition being described as comatose, we should expect the patient's hearing to still be intact because it was the last system to shut down. I thought I was being encouraging by telling her daughter that her mom could in fact speak, and that she did every morning. So, one morning the daughter came in to speak to her mother at 6:45. Her mother did not utter a word.

She never did speak to her family, and she died about 10 days later. There's a good chance I was the last person who heard her speak, and to this day, I have no idea why.

## Somebody's Sons

In the Surgical Intensive Care Unit, we cared for patients admitted for bodily trauma. Included were head injuries, post-operative open-heart surgeries, severe falls resulting in spinal cord injuries too severe for the neurology unit, gunshot wounds, etc. Not many things get to me as far as body parts and fluids. Not that I liked managing them or anything. But parts and fluids go along with the bodies of every living creature. Parts and fluids make us who we are as humans and are strong indicators of health or disease. It's preferable however, that said substances stay in their designated bodily locations, and parts remain intact.

One of two patients who touched me most was a young black man who had recently started a "good job" as an electrical lineman. Somehow, he fell, fracturing his neck vertebrae and making him instantly a quadriplegic. The fear, anxiety, disbelief, and sadness in his eyes as we took care of him, was heartbreaking. He was in his late twenties.

If that wasn't bad enough, I remember a white guy in his twenties who had been in a motorcycle accident without a helmet on, and who had sustained a skull fracture. Now, I'm very clear that wearing a helmet is not the answer 100 percent of the time. My brother's legs escaped further damage during his motorcycle accident, because the helmet was hanging on the side of the bike and absorbed the bulk of the impact.

But for this young man, the injuries proved fatal. After a few hours, he went into diabetes insipidus from the trauma. It was almost impossible to keep him hydrated; fluids were leaving his body that rapidly.

Shortly before my lunch break, the last indication that his injuries were fatal appeared. He'd had a craniotomy shortly after being brought into the ER that morning. While hanging yet another IV bag to try to keep up with the huge outpouring of urine, I noticed a thick, white substance oozing from the incision. By this time, the attending physician had come into the room to observe. "What's that?" I asked him. "Barb, that's brain tissue."

These two young patients impacted me tremendously. I tend to form connections with my patients and the two of them reminded me of my sons and the level of vulnerability I have as a mom because I could not, and would not, be able to protect them from everything. I had literally without wanting to, watched somebody's son lose almost all of his bodily fluid, as well as "his mind."

I was done for the day. No eating lunch, no talking, no nothing. Mic drop.

## Not From Housework

I was been somewhat of a wanderer. While working fulltime in my primary SICU (Surgical Intensive Care Unit), I always had a side job where I'd float across the city, checking out and working at other hospitals. It's called PRN nursing or working "as needed."

I really value experiences with different cultures and ethnicities, as well as in units with different staff. Through it all, patients were patients, didn't matter what skin color or gender. A disease was a disease. This didn't mean the disease process would not manifest differently because of the individual. It did. But it was basically the same and was identifiable. Most of the time.

There was a smaller, neighborhood hospital across town where I worked fairly regularly. It had a unit that wasn't quite as busy as my fulltime unit, but there were still interesting cases. I do not remember why this one gentleman was admitted, but while I was there, he was complaining of back pain. According to his history, he had been painting at home the prior weekend. He felt perhaps this was why the back pain. His blood pressure was dropping every hour or so, even though we were increasing his fluids. We knew something was not right.

The details are sketchy but after his BP dropped and him becoming pale and almost unconscious, I remember being told to draw an arterial blood gas level from the indwelling arterial line. An arterial line, or "art line" was usually inserted into the radial artery which is in the wrist. The tubing was then hooked up to a pressure monitoring system. When we saw the color of the blood that had been drawn, we were shocked! It looked as clear as cherry gelatin. That is NOT how arterial blood should look. The doctor immediately ordered a CAT scan and it was discovered the patient had a Triple A (abdominal aortic aneurysm) that had dissected (split open) and was leaking into the abdominal cavity. This was the reason for the up and down blood pressure, and the dilute blood.

Ultimately, the patient did not survive. An aneurysm that is already dissecting is major and gives a surgical team little to no time to address it. Dissecting abdominal aortic aneurysms have a 90 percent mortality rate. The one other dissected aneurysm patient I vividly recall was a patient in his forties who made it to and from surgery, then survived maybe nine months. He had a huge post-operative abdominal wound the size of a dinner plate that had to be packed with sterile moist gauze a couple of times a day. The wound-care process was intense enough; add to it the need for the patient to be up sitting in a chair once or twice a day and it was really a trip. It was not unusual for him to get up and half of the packing would shift and start falling out. It was terrible. Finally, he went to rehab, where he lived the last days of his life.

Sometimes I wonder why I have mild panic attacks, fretting about how myself and my sons are going to fare in life. Then I remember that my brain has plenty of these and other tragic memories, and I have to slow down and give thanks. But for the grace and mercy of God.

## The Ultimate Embarrassment

Culture, language and medical conditions have a tremendous effect on how individuals respond to their condition and to the caregivers trying to give care. There was an elderly German man admitted to our unit who only spoke and understood German and had a level of dementia. It's always good when you introduce yourself to the patient and tell them what you need to do. That's one of the first things we're taught in nursing school clinical rotations. This can involve actually touching them, changing an IV bag, emptying a urinary catheter, etc. With him, there were clearly limitations to communication.

Depending on how long the patient is on the unit, we individually may not know all that's wrong with them. We also may not know these things if they are not in the particular area of the floor that we've been assigned to cover. Short staffing can result in inadequate communication. Additionally, some basic care just needed to be done despite communication glitches. On this particular day, I was asked by another nurse to help her with this gentleman.

We greeted the patient by name when we went into the room and approached him, telling him we were coming in to make sure he was clean before lunch was served. As we pulled back the sheet, the man snarled and almost growled at us, violently tugging at the sheets to keep us from "exposing" him. The revelation was shocking.

The man did not have a penis. Actually, no external male reproductive organs at all. Instead, there was a small hole at the base of his perineal floor, that urine drained out of. I said DRAINED out of. This meant he had to be cleaned because there was no anatomical musculature that would allow him any control of urinary output.

As we age, "things" can happen. Our skin changes, joints, hair falls out, sexual function can diminish; and that's not even mentioning a variety of potential disease processes. Add to that issues of dementia and various types of trauma, including anxiety and stress over issues of daily living, and you've got a potential for a hot mess, to use another colloquialism.

Again, here's where I felt really bad for a patient. Being elderly, with a level of dementia, a language barrier and having a physical condition that quite likely in his mind, called his manhood into question, was too much for me to imagine. I will say this, though. For anyone who may be thinking how awful that was: consider women with mastectomies who have been going through this type of trauma for decades.

## Sweet Heart

Now, this one is more phenomenal than anything. I mainly worked at large teaching hospitals. That meant there could be a certain amount of research going on, and instances where we would see if a certain procedure, after careful consideration, would work. I have no idea who came up with some of those ideas, but it was NOT the nurses!

Let's fast-forward to what made me think of this particular experience. Recently, I was asked about a friend I grew up with and her post open-heart surgery status. Her chest had been left open after surgery. That's often done if there's swelling. It's not like you can just pull the stiches tight and close that chest up anyway. Many times, the swelling is indicative of infection. I told the inquirer "She'll be ight." (Please refer back to your handy 'Hood Glossary if you don't remember what "ight" means.)

An Open Chest Procedure was not necessarily uncommon, but it was still fascinating. "Wow!" I'd think to myself as I peered into the chest cavity at the beating heart and surrounding tissue. Now mind you, an open chest was probably the most sterile of sterile procedures that you'd ever want to prep for, outside of the OR. Sterile gown, head covering, gloves, goggles, etc. We looked like outer-space explorers!

In this instance, we used sterile 4x4 gauze pads, saline solution, and a Water Pik looking thingy, all sterile. I say thingy because that was a whole lot of years ago and I forgot what it was called. But that wasn't the clincher. The clincher was the five-pound bag of Domino sugar. That's right, granulated sugar, yellow and white bag, blue writing. The procedure involved (after suiting up) pouring a measured amount of sugar into the open chest cavity, letting the body fluids and heat liquify it over several minutes, rinsing it with sterile saline with the Water Pik® thingy, suctioning the now liquid, sugary syrup substance out with a sterile suction device attached to the Water Pik® thing, then lightly packing the cavity with the saline moistened 4x4 gauze. It took two of us to do this. This is one example of why it was imperative that all nurses on that unit, functioned on comparable levels. There were many things that we just could not do alone. That unit was a team, and we each had to be competent, accountable, and trustworthy.

As far as that sugary sweet procedure, why, you may ask, did we do all of that? Because someone researched and determined that it would be a good idea because the germs would feed on the sugar and not the patient's body tissues. Crazy thing is, it worked. After going through all of that in our unit, then going to the step-down unit, the regular floor, and finally being discharged home, the lady came back to visit, walking on her own, so we could see how well she was doing and to say thank you to us for her care.

For anyone who may be wondering, the patient was maintained in an induced coma while her chest was open. Can you even image the stress of being conscious and awake with all that going on? Jeez!

# 3 FIELD REPORTS: HOMECARE AND OTHER ADVENTURES

Besides schools and medical facilities, I've also provided services in homes, at the airport, in banks, law firms, private industries and factories, utility companies, governmental agencies like the Internal Revenue Service and Defense Finance and Accounting Services, your local fast food chain restaurant, and even given dialysis treatments on a cruise ship! Working in the field provides a different look at medical and nursing issues because it's not confined to areas where compliance can be monitored as closely. You'll see that in a couple of the stories. Field work as I call it, can also be fun! You'll see that, too!

Home care services are very important and play a large part in medical support. My role was to visit the clients' homes and make sure the client and the clients' families were satisfied, and the services were specific to the client's needs. My home care experiences were after my hospital nursing experiences. School nursing has been pretty much ongoing since leaving the hospital as well.

As far as facilities such as banks, the airport, etc., I've worked for a couple of EAP providers for many years. EAP stands for Employee Assistance Program. The general objective of the EAP is to ensure that employees get the support they need so they can function as close to 100 percent efficiency as possible on the job and at home. If the employee gets some support with day to day issues, it's felt the resulting peace of mind makes job efficiency easier. The EAP could help the employee with finding contractors, therapists, adult day care for aging parents and more. Sometimes I facilitate one- to two-hour brown bag lunch workshops on stress, time and change management and a variety of other topics. I also represent the company at corporate health fairs.

Then there is also what's referred to as Critical Incident Stress Management (CISM), situations requiring emergency emotional support at locations where a crisis has occurred. Incidents could be due to a death or some other significant trauma, affecting or involving the employees. Remember the Columbine shootings? That would be a CISM. So are local bank robberies during business hours. Counselors and staff members are dispatched to assist with grief, fear, shock, anger and disbelief. Sometimes the staff handles things well on their own, or with minimal assistance. Other times further support is needed.

## Clutter and Stuff

I did supervisory home care visits for about five years. I'm going to say this carefully so as not to be offensive. Some of our seniors have so much stuff that's been accumulated over the years, it's made me go home and start massively throwing things out. Then four months later, I would wonder to myself "Where's that pink vase? I thought I had one, now what am I going to put these flowers in?" That pink vase and a buncha other stuff had been ditched months ago in an anti-hoarding panic.

Some spaces were so cluttered it was like the client moved from a four-bedroom house with a basement and an attic, all of which are full of stuff, to a two-bedroom apartment with only a kitchen space and no dining room. Many of them probably did have to deal with downsizing like that. Once their physical condition starts to deteriorate, and when friends and family begin to pass on, what's left to hold on to are things. But, when I say stuff was everywhere, I mean exactly that.

There are some very real considerations for these situations. A client has the services of a HHA (home health aide), or an STNA (state-tested nursing assistant), who comes to help keep the house tidy, do light laundry, prepare some meals, and help the client with personal ADLs (activities of daily living) like bathing and washing hair. Assignments are pre-determined, and an agreement is signed. But that does not make the agreement easily binding.

Mrs. Johnson was a serious hoarder. There was so much stuff on her small kitchen counter, it was difficult to clean it. Boxes of cereal, bread, old dishes, pots and pans, and other random stuff. The same with the cupboards. The Brown Brothers were there, too.

Remember, this is Hood Medical. Brown Brothers is a hood term for roaches. The Brown Brothers don't care and will move in and invite all their friends and family members to come along, too. They can have a place on serious lockdown. Mrs. Johnson's apartment, especially her kitchen, was so full of stuff that it was not only difficult to clean, but the roaches had plenty of places to hide and reproduce. The nurse's assistant would be in tears. It was a difficult situation to correct because of Mrs. Johnson's chronic, physically debilitating disease process, and her very headstrong personality and angry disposition. Mrs. Johnson was not that old which was in part, why I think she was so angry.

I'm sure there will be many reading these pages who have various solutions to any number of the challenges and circumstances I speak of. Please keep in mind, in our society, there are laws in place, good or questionable, which can help or hinder. And if not laws? Then, privacy issues. Or choices. Rights. Family challenges. Greed. Denial. Disinterest. Family feuds. These situations can be complicated. Too bad, because while some families were at odds, the patient or client suffered. More.

## When Standing Was Deemed Best

Mrs. Williams' apartment regularly had the faint smell of urine. "Come sit down for a few minutes" Mrs. Williams would say smiling as I stood clutching my clipboard and pen tightly to my chest. ("Stop it!" I'd mentally tell myself. "She doesn't have roaches, it's the lady across town.") For some reason it felt like holding my belongings close to me would prevent one from getting on me.

"Oh, thank you, Mrs. Williams" I'd say smiling and using my most pleasant voice. "You know I've been traveling all over the city in that car and I'm tired of sitting. I need to stand and stretch for a minute!" Although I never wore anything that had to go to the dry cleaner, including coats, and although 80 percent of my overall wardrobe is from the thrift shop, I still could not risk sitting in damp urine, then transferring it to my car upholstery.

I know. Why did I assume that about the chair? It was because of the smell in the room and because of the large, dark, circular areas on the chairs. Remember: I was used to working in the hospital, specifically critical care units, where many patients could not talk. So, in part, we had to rely on our senses. My senses are heightened, especially smell. Odors can indicate infection, when a patient has soiled themselves, even blood has a distinctive smell. The odor didn't have to be from the chair, but I was not going to risk sitting in it. And urine or not, there's no reason to be rude.

Mr. Kovac's kitchen table on the other hand, was situated directly below his second-floor bathroom. There was a large, gaping hole in the ceiling with bits of moist, black fuzz around it. (OK well, mold.) The smell of urine was very prominent. It was obvious his house needed some serious repairs. Of course, I stayed away from being anywhere near the gaping hole in the ceiling. He eventually was able to get it repaired, thanks to a social service consult. I will not be able to reiterate enough in these pages, the fact that we never know how a person is living, or if they're simply surviving. My blessings, large or small, increase my level or gratitude, daily.

## Behind Closed Doors

For as many years as I've lived in my hometown, I never knew what types of things went on in the senior high-rise apartments that I drove by regularly. It's an interesting community. As much as one might be tempted to think the residents are old and senile, living in their apartments, sitting around doing little to nothing all day, for many, that is far from the truth.

Holiday time is celebration time. It's not uncommon to go into a building, up the elevator, and be greeted in the hallways by the smell of collard greens, chitlins and weed. Pardon me, collard greens, chitterlings and marijuana. What a wonderful smell! Not really, I hated that combination of smells. Just because you're older does not mean you want to give up your old habits. Many elders, or even people who are not elders yet, use marijuana for medicinal purposes, with good levels of success. But the recreational aspect continues, too.

Same for love affairs. A walker, wheelchair or cane, does not mean affection is a thing of the past. I encountered several "couples" on my visit list. They depended on each other and were a comfort. It was horrible when one of them died. Although, less than a month after one active, ninety-year-old gentleman's lady friend passed, he had another one. His rationale: he was too old to grieve for long. He didn't want depression and loneliness to set in. As they say in the 'hood, "I ain't mad at him."

There are plenty of seniors with grown children who need help. I found myself in the position of keeping the secret of young family members staying with seniors on a couple of occasions. Grown sons or daughters and their spouses and children, needing to stay in their parent's subsidized, one- or two-bedroom apartment because they're down on their luck. Although it's sometimes the case, it's not always because of negligence that people find themselves in bad situations. I'd hate to see my own children homeless and on the streets. Especially my grandchildren. That would probably bother me, or in these cases, my seniors, more than any ailment would, or would make the ailment worse. The problem in the case of my seniors was if the building management found out, they could lose their subsidy and be ordered to move. I knew what the deal was. But I minded my own affairs. There was no physical or emotional abuse going on that I could see. In one case, my client begged me not to say anything. I left it alone, knowing bad times don't last forever, and things change.

So, in recapping, let's just say, age does not necessarily limit sexual interest and activity. Some know how to, and do, work around limitations. Therefore, STDs are still possible. Marijuana is known to provide relief from pain and discomfort as well as insomnia, and finally, who's going to go into the homes of the elderly and police them? Just saying...

## Strange Pets as in, Rodents

A nurse co-worker told me this story a long time ago and I never forgot it. You never know what you'll encounter in someone's home.

"While doing a mother and newborn baby visit, I was setting out my equipment, in preparation for the exam of the mother, and lab work for the baby. Suddenly, out of the corner of my eye, I saw something scurry from one side of the room to underneath the couch that I was sitting on. I screamed and lifted my feet up. 'What was that?' The mom said, 'It's OK, that's my ferret.' 'What's a ferret??' I asked. It looked like a big rat, to me. She responded, 'a ferret is a cross between a squirrel and a rat.'

A rodent. A BIG one. I never worked so fast to complete the visit and make sure the paperwork all was in order, so no one else would have to endure what I had already endured!"

(Clearing my throat.) Plain and simple, I would've clowned up in there as in, acted a fool. Especially if I wasn't warned.

# Glaciers, Whales and the Midnight Sun

Included in my PRN options were calls to work dialysis. This meant orienting in the process to the degree that ultimately lead to my being offered a full-time position. Then after about 18 months, I got to go on an Alaskan cruise to provide dialysis treatments for some of the passengers. Dialysis is the process of cleansing the blood when a person's kidney function is insufficient to do so. Kidney function can deteriorate due to toxic substances such as drug abuse, or kidney failure due to a disease process like uncontrolled diabetes. Dialysis treatments are NOT TO BE MISSED. Most dialysis patients must be dialyzed three times a week, for an average of three hours each treatment. Many of them are young and active aside from needing the dialysis. Without these floating units, cruising would be impossible. Our work area was a ship suite, converted into a two-machine dialysis station, complete with tanks and tubing.

If you're thinking dialysis nursing automatically includes long-distance travel, that is not true. But, thanks to a company called "Dialysis at Sea" it most definitely can include travel. Do an online search of them. They specialize in providing dialysis services on select cruise ships.

There were two RNs and two dialysis techs. We had nine patients divided between the Monday-Wednesday-Friday group, and the Tuesday-Thursday-Saturday group. One tech and one RN would have them on the machine by 5 a.m. and completed by 9 a.m. The unit would be cleaned up within a half hour, and everyone would head out to enjoy a day in port, or a day relaxing on the deck if it was a day at sea. Cruisers came with their own orders, but there were also a couple of nephrologists available for emergency issues.

Anchorage was beautiful in July! There were more flowers blooming than I ever imagined, and I literally witnessed the midnight sun. The sun set in the early morning around 5 a.m., was down for about three hours, then rose again.

From the hotel in Anchorage, we went to Seward by bus to board the ship. I got to see glaciers as well as whales, but I did not get pictures of the whales. They were illusive when I was there. This was one of my most memorable and pleasant nursing experiences. All I had to do was get myself to Anchorage, and back home from Vancouver. The cruise and the amenities were payment for my services. I LOVE to travel, so it was a great trade-off!

## Smile for the Camera!

This experience was not hands-on nursing, but it reminds me of a saying I love "wherever you go, there you are." Nursing has been stable and wonderful, but I love frequent doses of the stage and performing, after which I can go home and chill in private. I am an artist at heart. Whether it's a script in a stage play or a monologue, singing, costuming, dancing or model talent for advertisements - I love the arts! So, wouldn't you know, when I was cast as talent in a promotional campaign for a large company in the medical field a couple of years ago, I was used as an on-site "consultant" of sorts, since I just so happened to be a nurse! "Go get Barb so we can see if we're doing this procedure correctly." How funny! I heard that all day and was happy to oblige. The casting guy had been clueless to the fact that I was a nurse. What a coincidence! I didn't even have to change clothes, despite bringing several outfits to the shoot.

It was almost business as usual, but with a fun twist and an opportunity for re-takes! Major difference from "real" nursing.

## Birds, Squirrels and Couches

Mr. Robinson was one of my favorite clients to visit. He was pleasant, jovial and loved nature, even living on the 10th floor of the high-rise apartment. I liked him in part because I too, am a nature lover. His balcony door was frequently open just a crack in case the birds he fed wanted to come in and pay him a quick visit. Or the squirrels. It was the story of the squirrels that got me.

I feed birds as well. I also leave something out for the squirrels on occasion. But squirrels must be monitored because they're bold and will take liberties if allowed. I'd occasionally leave peanuts out for them. All was well until one morning one of them smelled me roasting them. My living room window was open and the next thing I knew, that squirrel was spread eagle on my screen, looking in. I had to keep that window closed for a while.

Birds are beggars too, but "mine" are not to the extent where I let them in! I feed them two or three times a week. On some of the off days, they sit in the trees in front yard, looking into my living room, or they peck around the porch looking for food. Or, the blue jay will be out there on the banister yelling. Mr. Robinson, however, took it to a whole 'nother level, saying he occasionally and intentionally left a line of bird seed along the patio door sill to encourage them to come in. His friends the squirrels took it a step further, though. Several steps.

One day I was talking to the EMS (emergency medical services) crew in the hallway of his building. They wanted to know if he'd told me about the time two squirrels rolled up into his apartment and waited for him to come back from his errands. Mr. Robinson had trained those squirrels when they were young, to come in through the slightly open patio door. He showed them where their ONE peanut in the shell would be. They had to run over and jump up onto the folding chair, then onto the card table. He would coax them to take that one peanut by saying "go on, you know where it is."

A friend called to see if Mr. Robinson needed anything from the store. Mr. Robinson said he was bored and decided to go along. He left the patio door open and left his Medic Alert necklace on the same table the squirrels were used climbing onto in order to get their treat. You already know where this is going.

About a half hour after the building superintendent spoke to and witnessed him walking out the front door, EMS received an alert coming from Mr. Robinson's apartment. "But he's not here, I just saw him leave and I've been down here the whole time" the superintendent said. "Well, we legally still have to check it out" the EMS techs stated and all three of them got on the elevator.

If your guess was that the squirrels looking for their treat inadvertently set off Mr. Robinson's Medic Alert, you're right. They accidentally "called" EMS. When the superintendent and the EMS crew got into the apartment, one squirrel was on the table chillaxin, the other was laid out on the couch. They didn't hurry off, either. It's said that they took their time and had to be shooed out, probably thinking "Yo, where's our food, tho?"

Mr. Robinson decided to be more careful about leaving his patio door open. But he also said he made sure to offer his friends the squirrels, their treats as soon as he could, since he had "disappointed" them.

Creature shenanigans. Just, wow!

## Don't Move!

This story is from a long-time nurse friend who did quite a bit of skilled home care. I'm here to tell you, the aging process along with illness, can bring out a lot of behaviors and actions generated by fear, loneliness, anxiety, anger, regrets, abuse and who knows what all else. I can relate. That's why I do everything I think I want to and am able to do, within reason, while I can. That way, hopefully there'll be fewer regrets.

Mr. Smith was wheelchair bound. Mr. Smith was also used to having a gun in his home for protection. What I did not mention in my previous stories about home care for senior and disabled citizens is although the majority of caregivers are wonderful and honest people, there are plenty who are not. Theft and abuse are not uncommon. Many seniors do not appreciate having a stranger come into their home, invading their private space. They'd rather be able to do it themselves. Or not do it. I can't say I blame them, especially when they seemingly have no choice. Although many appreciate the help, many would prefer to continue to live life as they're accustomed to living it. Breaking years of old habits can be a real challenge, and combined with other issues, changing could be more than a notion. Decision making can be a difficult part of human nature across the board.

Apparently, Mr. Smith was used to defending himself in the past. Whatever all that meant to him, Mr. Smith had a loaded 45 caliber that he sat on while in his wheelchair. The reason he needed a skilled nursing visit was because he had a rather involved lower leg dressing that my friend had to kneel in front of him in his chair and change.

Again, going into people's homes means caregivers can encounter anything from the Brown Brothers, fleas, urine-affected furniture, rodents posing as pets, birds flying around, protective dogs, mean-spirited cats and God only knows what else. This is one reason why many of us working in home care, avoided pants with cuffs at the bottom, did not wear clothing that needed dry cleaning, left our purses locked in our cars and frequently stood for the visit unless we could be seated on metal or wooden chairs. While all of this might sound impolite, judgmental, holier-than-thou, paranoid or anything else, you would need to have followed us around for a few weeks so you could see why we took the precautions we did. Although in this book I'm talking about some of the less affluent, even impoverished, inner-city 'hoods, many of these same conditions do not discriminate based on race, gender, or socio-economic status. I feel it was much kinder to quietly take precautions than to be wilding out, running, screaming, tearing at clothing, smacking at things or anything else like that, in someone's house. I love to help, but I also know myself and my limits.

Mr. Smith was said to be a bit cantankerous at times. I think I would have come up with a rapid response plan on what to do in case of a meltdown on his part, too. A meltdown could come due to some level of dementia, and or could be related to carrying old, dysfunctional behavior into later years of life. But a discussion was had, and my friend told him very clearly, that if she even saw his hand move near that gun that he was sitting on while she was treating his leg, she would be sure to push him, and that wheelchair, over backwards.

She and Mr. Smith had an understanding and could laugh at it. They also kept it straight up 100% with each other. That scenario could have turned out badly on so many levels, but it did not, and I laughed out loud visualizing it. Sometimes nurses develop really strange senses of humor. It's almost like we have to in order to maintain sanity while we're in the trenches. Otherwise, it can quickly and easily become too much. We have to know our territory, know ourselves, and know our patients.

Not all patients receiving homecare services are angry or resentful. There are those who are lonely and appreciate visitors, wanting you to stay well past your designated time of service. Some will even resort to creating scenarios they feel will require you to stay. Homecare, just like any other nursing specialty, is an interesting, very unique aspect of nursing.

## Out and About

Nursing experiences are not only job-related. There've been several times where I found myself in the position to assist on the streets in the community. Shortly after I moved into my current home, I heard what sounded like falling on the front porch of the house next door. My neighbor who I had not met yet, was calling out to his friend, saying "Hang on man, I called the ambulance, they're coming!" When I got to the porch and introduced myself as the new neighbor, also a nurse, the man told me his buddy had a seizure and was having a hard time coming out of it. No emergency meds were available, so I waited with them until the EMS arrived, then went back home. I'd describe my neighbor as an orderly gentleman who listens to a kick-ass, old-school music playlist, loves working on old trucks, has at times put plastic flowers in his meticulously maintained yard, and rigs up sheltered areas on his front porch for the neighborhood's feral cats so they don't freeze in the winter. Most days, he simply gives me a nod of acknowledgement, except when I thanked him for rigging up lighting in front of my car and shoveling the front walkway. He said the backyard needed the light because it was too dark.

Then there are car accidents. I've stayed on at least two accident scenes, assessing conditions of those involved, encouraging them to be still and relax as much as possible, and reassuring them while waiting for emergency response. Thankfully, none of the accidents have been fatal.

Then there was the bicycle rider who was down in the snow, on the curb, as I was driving by. Both of my sons are avid bikers, so cyclists are special to me and I have a real problem with motorists who are inconsiderate, reckless or just plain don't care. Of course, there are certain rules cyclists need to adhere to, but too many motorists today are dangerous to themselves AND other car drivers, not to mention someone on a bike.

Unfortunately, it was at night and I was driving alone. The sad truth is, although we may want to help, sometimes we have to take another approach. There were several considerations: I could not tell if he was simply sitting down or if he was actually hurt, it was dark outside, and I was by myself. He seemed to be alone, but how did I know this was not a set-up with someone lurking or watching at a distance? There wasn't a lot of snow, but it was still cold. He was on his cell phone. Car-jackings are not uncommon. If someone assaulted me, I'd have been out in the cold, likely without a purse, phone or car.

If I don't consciously choose to take care of myself first, I cannot take care of anyone in need. I decided to call 9-1-1 and direct them to the site. They responded pretty quickly. A couple of miles down, I saw responders go by with flashing lights, in the direction of the biker.

All things considered, there's a saying I use all the time: "wherever you go, there you are." My nursing skills are good all day every day. I just have to use discretion.

Barbara J. Barrett

# 4 NURSING WITH CHILRENS

It was a huge change moving from critical care to working in schools. Initially, there was not a lot in the way of being "sick" as there should not be. I found myself making personal adjustments, and sometimes explaining to people, why I found a lot of what I saw working in the schools, to be trivial. Although those patients I'd worked with in the hospital were older and had medical diagnoses or trauma, the assumption of anything less being trivial was not fair on my part. I soon realized why it was not trivial and made the adjustment. In the case of children, I had to remind myself that not only is feeling bad relative and highly individual. It's also simply that: feeling bad, and children were still in a physical, mental, emotional and academic learning process.

Here are two examples. It's not unusual for children to arrive at school with a low-grade fever. But, a temperature of 101.2 degrees at 8:30 a.m. is something I would side-eye. It makes me wonder what happened or did not happen at home. I reminded children that parents should be made aware of any discomfort prior to leaving the house, and ultimately, it's the parent's responsibility to check the child before sending them to school. While I'm aware that parents need to be employed, it's not fair to knowingly send a child to school with a fever, and simply say "go see the nurse when you get to school." Some symptoms are obvious, but RNs are not licensed to diagnose. In my school district, we could not legally dispense medication without an order. Verbal consent from a parent is not the same as taking a verbal order from a physician, and the school setting is really different as far as protocol since there were no staff pediatricians. We certainly did not have x-ray or other detailed diagnostic equipment on site. Despite all this, I experienced children hurting themselves over the weekend and waiting until they got to school to address the issue with me because a parent actually told them to go see the nurse when they got to school. This is not acceptable.

Another example is children coming to school with a stomachache. The first likelihood is they did not have breakfast; the second is they are constipated. Either way, it's not a good start to a day of learning. For me, it can be very frustrating. Especially if the child arrives at school late, frequently, thus missing breakfast frequently. A lot of times, stomach aches are signs of anxiety.

Feeling bad can also be due to situations at home, causing psychosomatic symptoms. Why might a student arrive late to school regularly; why is it they do not eat breakfast most days and why would a parent not address an injury when it happens at home? It can be complicated to say the least. Because the teacher has a classroom full of students; because there may not be a psychologist full-time in the building; and because the likelihood of a social worker being readily accessible (if on staff at all) is nil, the nurse can become a catch-all. This is extremely frustrating.

There have also been a few times when I've reminded staff that because I'm the one who has the nursing license, I do not expect them to take time from teaching or administration, to assess or try to diagnose children's complaints, short of needing a bandage on a paper cut, or something minor like that. That would be like me trying to teach math. I'm not licensed to do it; it is not my job. This issue also goes the other way. A nursing or medical diagnosis coming from a teacher, as in telling a child what's wrong with them AND telling the child to inform the nurse of what they need, is a no-no. I'm sure many teachers know a lot, but no. Just no. Not like that, and not on the school's licensure-specific time, please. It may be done in an attempt to help out, and the staff comprises a team. But it's best to stay in our respective lanes. Now, if there's pertinent information, like a family history or a message from the family or other support staff, that's different and sharing can be important and helpful.

Over the last 15 years, there are more and more children with chronic disabilities and diseases in the public-school sector. Because of this, school nurses are a vital part of school staffing, particularly with younger children. Juvenile onset insulin dependent diabetes, tube feedings by way of MIC-KEY® buttons, urinary catheterizations, and ostomy care, are all justifications for licensed, professional, skilled nursing in more and more of our schools.

There are daily medications, PRN inhalers, EpiPens and seizure medication. Ideally, the parent, the student, the teacher and the school nurse become cooperative team members, so the child learns how to manage his or her condition, and classroom time remains as uninterrupted as possible. For many reasons, that can be a challenge.

There's also a newer trend of outside agencies offering services to students during school time. Mobile dentistry, vision teams offering free vision screenings and eyeglasses, nursing students from local nursing schools coming to do basic height, weight and blood pressure readings, and local hospitals coming with a mobile unit to do physical exams. While I think the idea of these services is wonderful, I also have concerns about: 1) disruption of classroom time, 2) the possibility of "relieving" parents of the responsibility for taking their children in themselves and 3) in the case of dental care for example, some kindergarteners experienced their first dental exam without a parent or close family member to guide and comfort them through it, which was not good. To expect the teacher, or even me as the nurse, to sit there and hold their hand when there's a school full of other children needing attention, is unrealistic, if not impossible. I just feel it is best if some of these first-time experiences are had with a parent. While I'm also aware that some single parents work and it could be helpful to have services at school, my experience is, many parents are unemployed.

In over 25 years of working as a school nurse in a large metropolitan area, I've seen a lot. During much of that time I've chosen to work as a substitute. Subbing allows me to travel the district and see all different races and ethnic groups of children and families. Kids are kids for the most part, aside from some cultural nuances. They're curious, funny, loving, and smart, but sometimes manipulative and angry. Most will keep it 100 percent honest with you, once they trust you. The following memoirs give you an idea of what a school nurse may go through on any given day. Some are amusing; some definitely are not.

---

---

# Back up Offa Me

If young children decide they like and trust you, or think you like them, they'll be all up on you. There is no personal space because they don't know what that means. What's your space is theirs. I've had children standing so close at my desk even, that their little arms or shoulders were touching me. Or they want a hug. Matters not if they're coughing, sneezing, or have wiped their nose on their sleeve. So, what? I guess in their minds the nurse should be immune to germs or getting sick. And I guess most of the time, I was.

When I'd take a year off from the schools in order to pursue other things and returned, I frequently caught some kind of flu-like bug. As long as I was in the trenches with the germs, I was good. Sometimes in a funny way, I had to say to the children "back up offa me! You're crowding up my space!" They'd smile and move away maybe three inches.

# Bullying

One reason children migrate towards anyone who they think will listen, is because of bullying. Bullying is something that makes me very angry because number one, it's hurtful and disruptive to those who are being bullied. The second reason is, if it's not checked and addressed effectively, there's a strong chance the bullying behavior continues into adulthood.

Childhood bullying can be a sign of a problem at home, with family members being at the root of a child acting out.

Bullying has gotten worse with the presence of social media and various electronic gadgets. Many parents are not aware that their children are on their cell phones and tablets late at night, way past the time they should be sleeping. Instead, they're texting and interacting through video with friends, and even with people they don't know. Most of the interactions are probably harmless, but even as a sub, children would open up to me about receiving mean-spirited messages, and even threats. That's where it starts to become problematic. One middle school student I worked with was so distraught over a social media situation, she was cutting herself.

Children need guidance, and unfortunately, many adults have dropped the ball. Video games and devices have become the new babysitters. Many young parents have their own messes going on with their devices and social media. Sometimes I wish we were "back in the day" again. Certainly, there were problems then as well, but easier access to more people behind a keyboard has made the bad, worse. The good thing is, parents who are on top of things and who are in co-operation with the school, still are in the majority.

Sometimes I have to encourage a child to talk to me and see what comes out, because "back up offa me" is not the thing to say, jokingly or not. In several cases, those talks have brought out things I really would rather not have known. But overall, my experiences with children have been rewarding, thought-provoking, adventuresome learning experiences, and wonderful opportunities to be of service, for which I am grateful. Without going into detail, let me just say that bullying occurs on several levels including cyber-bullying, direct bullying, indirect, destroying or damaging property, verbal and reputational, and on and on. This is not a small subject. There's still research going on about it. And please know, bullying is one of the reasons some of our children, particularly adolescents, are suicidal.

## Frequent Flyers

If children got travel miles for each trip to the dispensary they made, some would be able to go to Hawaii free of charge. I call them "Frequent Flyers." There is generally nothing whatsoever physically wrong with them. "Frequent Flyers" oftentimes have social or emotional issues. Or there are things going on at home making them uncomfortable, or even at risk. They could be fearful and simply need a space that feels safe. Or, they could hate math, not have done their science homework, don't read out loud very well so they want to avoid it, or they may be overweight and gym class is taxing to them. They could be being bullied, or they could simply not have the greatest of social skills.

Perhaps they're bored to death. They were curious and came in wanting to know what I was doing. Some of them hate tests. They went to bed too late. They're undiagnosed lactose intolerant and have regular stomach aches. They need eyeglasses (that's a later story). They have a toothache. They're immature and would rather be at home with mom, dad, the dog, the cat- anything but school. Or maybe they're hungry.

Whatever the case may be, I sometimes had to tell a child there is no reason why, after my only being at their school for a week, I should know them by name. While at school, their objective needs to be staying on task. I'd tell the older ones; school is preparation for having and maintaining a job. The priority at school is learning, and school is not a medical facility. Our employers expect there is a time to be on task at work, and a time to schedule appointments or take breaks. A certain level of order has to be demonstrated and taught for it to be understood. And a certain level of order helps encourage success.

## "I Wanna Stay Home Tomorrow. So, This What I'm Gonna Do..."

So, a mom came in one day with her first-grade son. "He thought he wasn't going to have to come to school today, but we fixed that." Child is mean-mugging and not talking. I was thinking to myself, "What's wrong with you?" Well, turns out, brilliant little dude got out of bed sometime during the night while his mom and siblings were asleep, went to the kitchen, and helped his allergic-to-peanut-butter-self to a nice spoonful of peanut butter. (Seriously, dude?) "If I have an allergic reaction, I can stay home!" This is what he thought because he was young, and his thought process was incomplete.

The fact that our children are thinking, but their thoughts are incomplete, can be dangerous. What he was not able to consider (because he was young) was: everyone was asleep in case he had a reaction, so he was on his own; if the reaction was severe, he could die; if someone did wake up and find him, he may not have to go to school because he may have had to go to the hospital. Fortunately, the spoon dropping into the sink woke mom up, and she gave him some Benadryl before the reaction really took hold. He turned out fine aside for some slightly itchy lips. I just looked at him.

It reminds me of the time I was at Girl Scout camp. I contracted poison ivy for the first and only time. It was very annoying. There was another girl there who had some emotional issues (somewhat DQ as in, drama queen) and she wanted to go home. So, she rubbed herself with poison ivy leaves, blew up like a balloon and was more miserable than she ever thought she'd be. This was a very fair-skinned white girl around 11 years old. Not only was she swollen the heck up, she was red and rashy. And miserable. Even back then, I just looked at her, too.

## A Plethora of Needs

"Miss, do you have…?" "Nurse, can you…?" The following is a partial list of things children and staff have come to ask school nurses for, and some situations we have been asked to address. Trust me when I say I'm not making these up. I have no reason to. We just need Superwoman T- shirts, that's all.

- An apple (or other fresh produce)
- Something to drink (other than water)
- A sandwich (Seriously? An entire, freshly made sandwich??)
- A pencil
- Pencil sharpener
- Contact lens solution (You're pushing it, now.)
- Eyeglass repair kit (OK, a lot of us do.)
- Notebook paper
- A blank CD (C'mon now. I'm a singer, but really?)
- Something to substitute as dental wax (for wearers of braces) because student forgot theirs
- Duct Tape® (See explanation below.)
- Nail polish or eye makeup remover
- Salt, pepper, and or sugar

- A quarter
- Socks
- Underwear
- Migraine headache pills (requested by a third grader with no diagnosis)
- Chapstick
- "Can you get this eyelash outa my eye?" (It's lying inside the bottom lid. A clean, wet, cotton-tipped swab will get that out.)
- "There's a popcorn kernel stuck up her nose..." (brought down by teacher)
- "A pencil eraser is in his ear..." (brought down by a teacher)
- "There's a ring (as in, a piece of jewelry) stuck in her throat..." (brought down by teacher)
- "She has a bird feather stuck in between her teeth that I watched her pick up off the ground..." (Brought down by teacher. Lil girl, what were you thinking?)
- "This itching inside this cast is driving me nuts and I can't concentrate in class..."

Now, this right here is where it really gets 'hood because I was looking at half of these questions and scenarios like, WTH? Seriously? I can understand something to drink, and maybe the apple. We'd take leftovers from the cafeteria for diabetics with hypoglycemia, as well as to give to students who have not eaten breakfast or who need a snack. A sandwich was pushing it. Salt and pepper kind of was, also. Maybe the salt is reasonable, because some of us use it as a gargle with warm water for children with sore throats. But there are times when I've had to remind those chilrens that my dispensary is not Walmart, or some sandwich joint.

As far as contact lens solution? I can understand. They don't know the tip of the dropper needs to be sterile, or at the very least, only used by one person. Teachable moment. The eyeglass repair kit? Maybe.

Then there was the time I had to rig up something to help a student with new braces until he brought his wax in. If you've had braces, you know the inside of your mouth has to get used to that metal. You also know you have to be very careful about substances that can get caught up in the metal and other tiny workings of the braces. What I ended up doing was wetting a cotton ball and tying it inside of the finger of a glove, cutting it down to about the size of a quarter, flattening it, and giving it to him to hold in his mouth between his teeth and the inside of his mouth. It was a good substitute. Jeez.

Wanna know what the Duct Tape® was for? That request was from a teacher. It was because the top of a student's shoe had come apart from the sole and was flapping in the wind. I taped it together. Why do I do these things instead of calling a parent? Well, I do call parents for many things. For others, I just manage it with as little disruption as possible. But, as an aside, parents? If your phone is off and it's not a dire emergency, I don't always have time to go through every emergency contact number you gave me, only to come up with all of them disconnected. This is NOT a rare occurrence. It's frequently the case across the district. While I can sympathize, it's very frustrating as well as unsafe. And it can also mean, your child may come home with their shoe being held together by Duct Tape®.

I'm sure some of you are wondering why the teacher sent the shoe repair issue to the nurse. Well, it's probably because I had a couple of different kinds of tape, even though I'm sure the custodian had some as well. Quite honestly, had I been the teacher, I probably would've tried the nurse first too. Or the art teacher. I thought that one was kind of funny.

Now, let's skip past the requests for items, to those incidents. The bird feather incident was a first-grade girl. Picked the feather up off the ground before school, and for some reason, decided it would make a good toothpick, I guess. Funny thing was, when the teacher brought her in, the student had her lips tightly sealed shut. I asked her to open her mouth and she cracked it open just enough for me to see this wet, fuzzy-looking thing sticking out slightly. I couldn't believe it. I pulled it out, gave her mouthwash, and asked her to please refrain from using bird feathers off the ground from random bird backsides, as toothpicks.

Then there was the teacher who brought in a third-grade student who had a pencil eraser stuck in his ear canal. I could see it, but it was in too far for me to try to get it out. The sight of it in there was driving me nuts, but I knew not to fool with it. His mother was at home feeling under the weather. She was fit to be tied when I called her to come get him because he HAD TO go to the emergency room. I told him his mother was not happy, and if I saw his hand go anywhere near his ear, I'd cut his hand off. He was crying because he thought they were going to have to cut his ear off in the ER. I told him I'll bet he wouldn't put anything else in his ear.

One of my coworkers had a student who, for what the heck ever reason, put a popcorn kernel up her nose. Luckily, she was finally able to blow it out. Potential choking and breathing hazard.

And how about the one who had to go to the ER because she

had a ring, as in a piece of jewelry, in her mouth and accidentally got it stuck in her throat. Kindergartener. The good thing in this case was it was not fully obstructing her airway because of the open nature of a ring, so she could still breathe.

Now, about the child who came in with itching up under his cast- I can relate. I broke my ankle when I was an eighth grader. The itching down in that cast almost drove me nuts some days. At the time, I did not know what I could use to scratch and relieve the traumatized skin that was getting very little oxygen and no soap and water. Before I go any further, here's another disclaimer. I am NOT advocating the use of ANYTHING to scratch in there. Ask your doctor for suggestions, whether it be a device, meds or something else. I know itching inside a cast is obnoxiously annoying but unfortunately, I had to send the student back to class with no solution. A pencil? No, the lead may break off. A cotton-tipped swab or those thin wooden stick thingys we use to part hair when we're chasing lice? Nope, same thing, they're brittle. Plus, we don't want anything that might be hard enough to scratch the skin or push on the mending bone and tissue. And no ink pen because it may leave ink on the skin and cause irritation.

But that straw cleaner I got from the houseware department at a local department store? Hmm. REALLY thin, fine metal, soft brush, and pliable!

I'm rarely surprised at what children do, or the needs they come in with. But, some of them are still *"SERIOUSLY Y'ALL?"* moments.

## Lucy and the Whiners

I needed to go to the kindergarten classroom. It was Monday

morning and Mr. Mike was covering for the regular classroom teacher. You would think on Mondays, children would come in refreshed and ready to learn, not a care in the world. Um, no. I'm not sure why, but many of them come to the dispensary to see the nurse within the first hour of arrival. Some even come straight out of their parents' car. Like Lucy.

(The date was November 10. Please remember this small fact because it'll be pertinent later in this story.) "What's wrong, Lucy? Why do you have that look on your face?" "I'm sick!" she said with high-pitched whining and forced tears. "Tell me what happened. Do you live with your parents? Did you tell them you're sick?" "I live with my mom and dad. I told them" "How did you get to school?" "My dad dropped me off." Lucy's temperature was normal; I saw no notation in the computer of chronic illness and no other outward signs and symptoms. And the crying had stopped, and she was looking around at things in the dispensary. "My goodness Lucy, you mean to tell me you told your dad you were sick, and he dropped you off here anyway?" "The doctor said I had pneumonia." "Really? When was this?" "In the summer." (Girl, bye. Remember, it was November 10 at the time of this story.)

So, after a talk and a bit of orange juice, I took Lucy by the hand and walked her back down to the classroom. Children are so cute! Five-year-olds who'd only been in kindergarten a couple of months, and who luckily didn't know me from Eve. I told Mr. Mike Lucy appeared to be fine. He then told the class to say good morning to the nurse. *NO*, I was thinking to myself! My cover will be blown, *DON'T TELL THEM I'M THE NURSE!*

Too late. Now Mr. Mike's darling little chilrens were tuning up into a sob-story symphony, whining their little heads off about aches and pains they've had or imagined since birth. I politely slipped out, leaving Lucy and the Whiners, behind. Poor Mr. Mike.

But Lucy and the Whiners had a nice, artistic ring to it!

## The Fragrance of Musk

Walking out of the dispensary and into the hallway, I could smell it. I know skunk odor because we lived in a neighborhood where skunks were common, and as a child, I used to go away to camp in the summer.

The second-grade boy walked in, pale and somber looking. "We have an issue with skunks at our house," he said. Those were his exact words. As I found him clean clothing, he told me there were skunks living under his front porch and sometimes they would spray, and it would get in the front closet where some of their clothes were kept. I thought his language was odd for a second grader. But whatever the case, he could not sit in class like that.

While he was in the bathroom changing, I called the social worker to ask if there was anything that could be done to assist the family. Perhaps they needed help in getting and paying for an exterminator. She said she'd look into it.

When he came out of the bathroom, he gave me a hug and went to class. I felt bad for him because he looked miserable.

On another occasion, a student came to my office first thing in the morning, crying. She said her dog had gotten skunked the night before, and now she smelled like skunk. She was crying because the other children were laughing at her and covering up their noses with their clothes. She said her older sister smelled like skunk, too. I told her it wasn't their fault, and about how our dog had gotten skunked years ago when my sons were in school. We were able to smell skunk in the air, and he was outside. He was young and goofy. We caught a whiff of him before he got in the door. Yep. Caesar had been skunked.

I shared with her how for the next hour or so, we washed him outside in canned tomatoes with the juice, tomato paste (we didn't have any plain tomato juice), Pine Sol, vinegar, bar soap and water and anything else we could find. Steam was coming up offa him as we scrubbed him down, because it was chilly outside. He had a guilty, miserable and sheepish look on his mug, and his ears were pinned back like dogs do when they know they've messed up. We did a pretty good job with the cleaning! He was able to come back in smelling like tomato and menthol.

These girls' father had just gotten off working the night shift. Mom was already at work. We did not have extra clothes in the girls' sizes at the school, so he had to come and get them. He arrived with the baby brother who looked to be about six months old. Dad said he'd had to open all the windows and turn off the heat. I could only imagine because the skunk smell was noticeable in the school lobby, from the short time they were in there. Poor children, poor pooch and poor dad! The things people go through! But, kudos to dad for handling it!

There are days when I admittedly have my own issues at the forefront of my mind, and I seriously wish things would just be business as usual at work. No "extra" or "over-the-top" issues, as the young folks call them. For me, business as usual outside of work is for the most part, peaceful, pleasant and productive; I'm free to go and do what I want, and I have a life. But there are way too many children and families who have too much to deal with, even families who society would consider to be stable.

Life.

## Children and Diabetes

I have my theories about why the increase in juvenile onset insulin dependent diabetes type 1. I do not recall diabetic children being prevalent when I was in school in the same district. In nursing school, we had to rotate through the pediatric specialty unit at a neighboring city's children's hospital. The pediatric patients who have left the greatest impact on my overall nursing career are those who've been diagnosed with insulin-dependent diabetes.

The newly diagnosed younger children can still be very silly despite having just been diagnosed and hospitalized with blood glucose levels of over 600. That's because they're too young to comprehend the seriousness; the intravenous fluids and insulin make them feel better and they're still children. But, when it was injection time, the whole silly vibe understandably changed.

Convincing them to stick themselves with even that tiny needle was a trip. The whining and procrastinating would start up, oftentimes followed by tears, and even anger and refusal. Eventually with most, we'd have to give their hand a gentle push.

I can relate. When I worked the diabetes camp, the attending physician required us to inject ourselves with saline during staff orientation. It took me the longest time to push that needle in!

We had to do it so we could understand what it felt like. It makes little difference that insulin needles are what I call "mosquito bite" needles. They're still a needle and they still stick you. Even in nursing school, some of our instructors had to give some student nurses a boost when giving that first patient injection.

Children must adjust to being diabetic, and all of the things that go along with it. This includes good food choices, calculating carbohydrate intake and insulin doses, and regular blood glucose level monitoring. It's hard enough for adults. We had a nurse in one of the critical care units who was very overweight, ate anything she wanted and would simply check her blood glucose level, and give herself doses of insulin. I know of other adults who don't check their blood sugar levels for weeks and eat whatever, only to end up in the hospital with levels over 700. Denial is an awful, potentially dangerous thing. It's necessary to help the students and the families get past the anger, shock and denial, so they can maintain a good level of health despite the diagnosis.

Camp Ho Mita Koda, the diabetes camp in Northeast Ohio, is a wonderful place for diabetic children and teens to go to have a great time with other children who are diabetic. Most of the counselors are former campers with diabetes. It was a blessing and a priceless learning experience for me to work there several summers, even though I am not diabetic.

One of my most memorable and amusing experiences besides playing pirates in the small lake, was going on a slicker hike. It was my first or second day there, having come after the rest of the staff. It seemed like it had been raining for 10 days straight, and the ground was a sopping, muddy mess.

Well, I was one of the designated nurses to go on the hike that day. This was an all-camp activity and there had to be two or three nurses in attendance. I knew I was in trouble when we had gotten maybe 10 feet into the hike and the 12-year- old boys were picking up hands full of mud and throwing it at each other. Of course, it got on staff, too. Becoming a muddy mess was part of this hiking process. It didn't help that I had to carry a large tackle box full of supplies. And I kinda was not in the position to protest.

The next thing I knew, we were going down into a ravine. It was one of those areas I thought of as uncharted territory. I would never in my life have thought of going down there. Why, there could be all kinds of creatures in that brush, mud and small tributaries of water! Plus, it was slippery. I was starting to become annoyed at having to lug that tackle box and not use my hands and arms to brace myself. But then, my hands would have been really disgusting, and could have possibly touched a creature. I like to look at and marvel over creatures, but not touch them, especially unexpectedly!

I was glad I had on my water shoes, but my reliance on and confidence in my water shoes soon changed once my shoe and foot got stuck in mud that was midway up my calf. It felt like my leg was in a suction device, being sucked down into what, I didn't know. Suppose I couldn't get it out, I thought. What if I sank deeper like I saw people on TV do when they got into quicksand? I had to very carefully take the shoe off, or risk losing it. I could see nothing but mud. All I could think of was the possibility of leeches attaching to my leg; those blood sucking wormy things that lived in muddy areas just like what we were voluntarily hiking through. But I couldn't lose my mind and start screaming and running because there was nowhere to go except into more mud that God forbid, I might fall into with the tackle box and all those syringes, insulin vials, glucose tabs, etc.

Climbing would require a level of calm if I were to be afforded the opportunity to escape. But then, I kind of couldn't escape because that would mean I would fail miserably, and the children would think I couldn't possibly save them from unforeseen dangers, let alone help manage their diabetes. After about two minutes, I pulled my bare foot and the shoe out, and was able to continue walking. I didn't even look at my foot to see if there were leeches on it. I just didn't want to see it. The kids, especially the boys, were watching me smiling, no doubt deciding if I was passing the test. I had to maintain my cool!

As we continued walking in the ravine, we got wetter and muddier. Did I mention it was still drizzling and children were still throwing mud at each other, large glops of it narrowly missing my face, but catching bits of my locs? Silly me, I should have wrapped my hair up, but I'd had no clue as to what was about to happen.

Finally, after what seemed to be an eternity of struggling through 10 miles of mud (an exaggeration), we got to the lake where we were able to rinse off. Seriously y'all? This was too much! It's a good thing it was close to 90 degrees outside. I had to quickly rinse my arms, legs and feet, in waters where fish, turtles and probably snakes swam free; then run back to the main hall dispensary, still hauling the tackle box, so I could disinfect my arms and hands, and prepare to count carbs and draw up insulin. Playing pirates in the lake was one thing. But "cleaning off" in there, then sitting in the dispensary like that, was quite another.

Hair with specks of mud in it, clothes damp, uncertain as to what mud dweller might be stuck on me someplace. I couldn't *WAIT* to get done and go shower. *BUT* I passed the test with the kids! I could hang!

The children's numbers were well controlled because the whole purpose of the camp was to have a safe, supportive, fun place where they could have fun with other diabetic children. The timing of blood glucose checks, carb counting, insulin administration, meals and food choices, and activities, were all focused on their needs.

The public-school system is a different story. Whereas schools used to be able to function just fine without a school nurse, with the rise in juvenile onset diabetes and the influx of more and more children with other special/skilled-care needs, qualified nursing personnel is necessary. When I attended school in the same district, I only saw the nurse at a distance once in 18 years, and she was doing paperwork.

Although most diabetic children I've encountered are pretty well adjusted, resistance to the whole idea is understandable. They don't want to have to go to the dispensary and check blood sugars, they aren't feeling having to be bothered with insulin whether by injection or pump, and they certainly don't want anyone telling them what they can't or shouldn't eat. Since they're young and have not had diabetes for 20 years, they generally feel OK because they have not developed the complications or negative side-effects that can develop due to years of mismanagement.

One nine-year-old student had what I called "suppliers." Other children would bring him plastic zipper bags of donuts, cake, cookies, candy, all sorts of carby, sugary stuff. We tried to shut that down, but doing so with determined children and lax parents, can be a real challenge. Or parents who feel that they can just let the child eat anything they want and give them as much insulin as is "needed." No. Good dietary habits must be taught. Many of our students learn to do very well, but too many do not, or they rebel.

I've had to be creative. Like, telling a younger student who was having eating and compliance issues that I was going to smell his breath after he ate to see if it smelled like candy and sugar, or lunch food. He believed I could smell a difference, which I could. He also thought it was so funny, he'd come up to me smiling, saying "My breath smells like lunch today!" But this tactic would not have worked in the following scenario.

There was an eighth-grade student I'll call Candy Mouth. I worked with Candy Mouth off and on from the time he was in kindergarten with newly diagnosed diabetes, to the time he graduated and moved on to high school. During that last year, he became more careless, in part because he was hanging with a shady crowd of young men. The good thing was despite his noncompliance, he and I were on good terms. I became tired of his blood glucose level being 400 or more upon his arrival to school in the morning. Based on my experiences, I would prefer blood glucose levels for younger elementary school children during school hours to range around 150. Yes, that's a bit elevated, but they're active, busy bodies, constantly moving, running, jumping, pinging off the walls, may be scheduled for gym or outdoor recess, and they can drop very quickly. If the levels get too low and they become lethargic, that's not a good thing. But 400 is a serious no-no, and he was 13. According to his mom, he'd only have about 40 grams of carbs for breakfast, and he had his insulin. He denied having anything to eat on the way to school. I was going nuts with him and knew he was eating something. Good thing was, he and I still had a good relationship and he would hear me out, even if he didn't comply. This was important!

One day the security guard came in and gave me a handful of candy that he had confiscated from Mr. Candy Mouth upon entering the school that morning. "I thought you might need to see this." YES, thank God for some evidence! I took it home and said nothing for two days.

Let me stop here to make a point before sharing the rest of this story. In my experience, key people need to be aware of a child's diagnosis. The security guard was a key player in turning this scenario around.

On the third day, with a blood glucose level of 423, I very calmly said to him "Wow, your blood sugar is so high! And guess what I have at home that Mr. Warren the security guard gave me? A hand full of Squirrels® and Now and Laters® he confiscated from you the other day. You know what confiscated means? It means he took them from you because you weren't supposed to have them." Dude didn't say anything, was just looking at me like he knew he was busted. "You know what?" I said to him "This is serious on levels that you may not even know yet, because you're young. But, remember telling me about that new girlfriend the other day?" With this, he started smiling ever so slightly. I leaned in and smiled ever so slightly too, and said "well, the problem with those really high blood sugar levels is that over time, if you're not careful, your 'stuff' won't work." Dead silence and you should have seen the look on his face.

Now, I know there's going to be someone who reads this and is going to think how awful, out of line or crude it was of me to say this to him. But I kid you not. His levels started going down significantly, almost immediately. At 13 years old, the unfortunate truth is, many of our children are sexually active. That's why there's STD education. So, if he can be educated about STDs, I could and did tell him about the possibility of his sexual function being affected due to uncontrolled diabetes. I would not have told that to any of my eight-year-old diabetics or even some of the 12-year olds who are not at the same level socially as Candy Mouth. Sex is a normal fact of life, and for him, so is diabetes. I knew him, his numbers had become dangerously high, we had a rapport, he was in his early teens and he was bragging about a girlfriend. I would do whatever worked within limits. Children do not always take advice from their parents as readily as they will from someone they trust and don't live with, especially adolescents and teens. Diabetes does not have to be a death sentence, nor does it mean as a young man, he could not have a healthy, happy life including sexually, and even have children. It's about management. These are things many medical practitioners unfortunately do not share with their young patients.

Let me take a moment real quick to talk about simple management. One of the first things that needs to be taught is label reading. All foods have nutrition labels required by the FDA (Food and Drug Administration), except some meats, and some prepared foods like deli salads. Meats generally have no carbs unless mixed with other ingredients, and oftentimes other foods nutrition content can be obtained online, or by asking the store or restaurant for the information. We have to share this information with families and students so they can be proactive.

The next consideration is we here in the good old U.S. of A. have portions way larger than the general half cup standard, so that needs to be taken into consideration. Also, a good portion of the liquids we drink are loaded with sugars which translate to carbs. This includes "healthy" fruit juices, which is why they're frequently used to correct a low blood glucose reading.

One way to help in carb control is to encourage diabetics to develop an appreciation of water. Water has zero carbs and will help bring an elevated blood glucose level down. While I'm not diabetic, nor am I a dietician, like most families who are faced with diabetes, research and medical advice are needed. My knowledge base comes from both. Caring for numerous diabetic children and adults, and interacting with their doctors, nurse practitioners and families has provided me with enough standard information to pass on, as well as to use for myself and suggest to diabetic friends. Certainly, in situations where blood glucose levels are well above or below normal, and when maintaining a certain level of nutrition along with those levels is a concern, you want to consult with and be assessed by your healthcare professional. A dietary consult is also a good idea.

Finally, I've met a few parents who have just not been able to accurately count carbohydrates and calculate insulin dosages. This could be due to mental or intellectual limitations, stress, depression, distraction, the parent's own personal issues, issues with other siblings or even anger due to having a child who requires this level of care. Whatever the reason, the child must be taught to be self-sufficient over time and this becomes a huge part of the school nurse's role. It's not easy because what's not enforced at home makes it that much more of a challenge to enforce at school, but it's not impossible! Dietary and nutrition training are a part of the diabetic management process and are offered to families of diabetic children in the hospital setting. But it's not always used to the fullest, nor is it always comprehended. I hate when any of my children are hospitalized for a reason that could have been prevented.

## Special Education Considerations

In addition to the diabetics, there are numerous children who for various reasons, cannot eat like the rest of us, who are unable to urinate on their own due to medical issues, who may have ostomies that need care, and who require dressing changes. Add to that, ADHD and ADD medications, severe allergies that require EpiPens to be on hand, inhalers and or nebulizer machines for asthmatics, and injectable medications for seizure control.

Most of the students and parents dealing with special needs, function effectively through teamwork with the school and community. Some have severe autism, many are non-verbal, and some children have behaviors dangerous to themselves and others. All children require supervision, but some special needs children require a much higher level. They cannot be told what to do, then left to follow directions. Their parents can be young, single women or men, who would love to have a normal life. But if their children are wheelchair-bound, non-verbal, and cannot feed or toilet themselves, it can create physical, social and emotional challenges. There may be a grandmother or other responsible adult who is available to and will help, but sometimes there is not. Sometimes the assistance is left up to an older brother or sister. While in many cases I've seen levels of family cooperation work nicely, I'm also aware of others resulting in major problems. I have been told by a couple of parents that extended family members have clearly stated they would help with the "normal" siblings but want no parts of watching the special needs child. In defense of those who will not take that responsibility, I'm not going to assume it's out of malice. There could be legitimate concerns about not being able to handle the child's needs effectively, resulting in further problems. I really don't know what to say to mothers who cry when they're repeatedly called to the school due to issues with their special-needs child. I don't know what that experience is like, and I'm not going to potentially trivialize it by saying things like "Oh, it'll be alright!" or "Don't worry, God is good all the time!" I don't walk in their shoes and I'm quite clear that I do not have any idea what it's like. I leave work and go home where I get a break from it all until the next day. Usually, I'm just a listening ear. I may ask questions about whether they've considered options for help that I may be aware of. Social service agencies may also be able to help by suggesting options. Special ed staff, physical and occupational therapists, teaching staff and nurses are trained to do a lot of things. But ultimately, final responsibility, whether it be actual hands on or administrating over their child's care, lies with the parent/guardian or caregiver, 24 hours a day, seven days a week.

What a very intense life it must be. Especially for parents in their twenties. My heart goes out to them. Some have figured out how to handle it very well. For others, it's a continuous struggle. And for some, it's a nightmare.

Considering all of this, several years ago, the county where I live not only began to close the doors of their special-needs schools for children, they also started closing the sheltered adult workshops for adults with disabilities. The children were "mainstreamed" into the public-school systems. When I asked why the adult workshops were being phased out, I was told it was because of the shift to promoting what's called "employability." I can't talk to you about the specifics of employability, but my concerns are for the adults with special needs, and their aging parents.

The county sheltered workshops provided numerous mentally and physically handicapped adults with daily supervised activity and work. A lot of the work was simple: sorting screws, nails, and other hardware items. They would earn a small paycheck. There were mental health staff workers there to monitor and assist. Many of the handicapped workers were in their thirties, but some were in their fifties. That meant their parents could be seventy years old, or more.

I was told in five years or so, we could expect the facilities to be closed. Summer services to special ed children are also beginning to be cut and eliminated. What I'm going to say next, I hope will be received in the manner intended.

I've had many years of working with special needs children. Once again, there are many levels of functionality. Some will never be able to do anything themselves, including chew and swallow food. There are others who cannot walk, but their brains are fully intact. Some have sleep issues. If the needs are significant, the individual affected cannot be left alone. They are a danger to themselves and others. They don't know any better. They cannot be left in bed, unrestrained, with the bedroom door open so they can come and go to the bathroom at night if they need to. Some children are climbers, and some will even leave the house at night. Remember the earlier story of the "regular ed" child who got up and purposely ate the peanut butter he knew he was allergic to?

I wonder if those responsible for making the decisions impacting people's medical lives, are fully aware of the impact of their decisions? What about the aging, 60 years old and older parents, particularly those with health issues, who have a special needs grown son or daughter? What are they expected to do? What can be done? Especially if they are not financially well off, or don't have property that can be attached in order for them to pay for assisted care or residential living? What are we doing here in the US?

Like the young folks say, I'll just leave this right here.

## Special Education Issues and Parental Denial

In consideration of the previous paragraphs, I'm sure the path to recognizing and accepting that one's child has mental or developmental challenges can be very difficult. There are many parents who are in denial, and who lose valuable time getting help for their children. There is no good reason I can think of for a typical four-year-old student to regularly yell, scream, cry, and hit strangers if she's not subdued and placated. While waiting to be picked up and taken home, she gets angry with everyone who walks in the door who is not her parent. At home, the parents admit to allowing her to stay up watching television at all hours of the night, and to giving her coffee. She spends the day sleeping in the classroom while the other students work. She requires a one-on-one classroom assistant because of her volatile behavior. Her parents think her behavior is fine and do not want her evaluated. Although the classroom she's in is a special needs classroom, sleeping is not what the rest of students do, nor is their behavior combative. Many are there due to developmental delays or cognitive challenges, both of which can result in a child testing a bit behind their peers.

Many times, the parents of special needs children have difficulties themselves and would benefit from a third -party advocate. That is, if they would accept one. Unfortunately, it is not uncommon in these situations, for the parents to lose custody. But even that takes some time because they too, have rights. It can also further traumatize everyone involved, making matters way worse.

My questions include, what about the child's right to services in a timely manner? What if he or she is taken away from her parents because of what the county may perceive as neglect? It's not that the parents don't love the child. It's that sometimes their way of showing love includes permissiveness and sharing coffee. Taking away custody is not the first, nor always the best answer. But at this rate, what are they going to do when she turns 13? Or 25? Is she going to be able to take care of herself once she's grown? Or will she grow up and continue the same cycle or worse, with her own children?

I do not have the answers to this situation. Mental health resources and social work are not my specialty, and the nature of mental health issues vary. But, do we understand this is one of many reasons why outside agencies and the government end up taking control of people's children and families? I want people to know what's going on and think about it. ALL families have someone (or several "someones") with some form of mental or emotional health issues. One thing I do know is, family needs to advocate for family, and beyond that come workers suggesting expert services. That includes nurses; social workers; physical, occupational and speech therapists, school psychologists, and anyone else who can point those in need in the right direction.

Really, what is our society going to do? The abundance of mental and emotional health challenges makes even voting for legislators and public issues, for example, that much more important.

Food for thought.

## Head Challenges

Young children are often plagued by what I consider to be childhood nuisances. I remember one child having head ringworm to such a degree that the affected scalp began to swell. My recommendation to the family was to take him to the doctor for immediate treatment. Ringworm can damage hair follicles and stunt future hair growth, leaving small bald areas. The family for whatever reason did not take the child to be assessed. This was right before Christmas break. Over the break, they finally took him, and he was hospitalized and put on IV medication. My guess was the doctors were probably concerned about the family's ability to comply with treatment at home since it had progressed to that degree. The student's hair loss was significant. Ringworm, especially of the scalp, is fungal and needs to be treated immediately. As much as I wish the topical, over-the-counter ointments were sufficient to cure it, they are not beneficial to scalp ringworm. A doctor or other medical practitioner must be seen to prescribe treatment.

Then there's head lice. Lice have been around for centuries and are not going anywhere. The American Academy of Pediatrics (AAP) states that head lice are not an indication of poor hygiene. They are a nuisance, not a health hazard. Therefore "No healthy child should be excluded from or miss school because of head lice and 'no nit' policies for returning to school should be abandoned." This policy and the accompanying article are dated June 26, 2010. Its why many school district policies have changed as far as exclusion for lice. There is no exclusion except in maybe rare, extreme cases. Maybe. You can check it out online. So, nope. Nurses nor teachers made up this statement, nor the resulting policies. Doctors did and school systems have the option to adopt it.

Meanwhile, parents absolutely hate being told their child has lice. To many, having lice is a social stigma. It's always someone else's child who is responsible for "bringing" lice into the classroom and "giving" them to their child. But lice can come from many places. For example, the backs of public chairs, especially plush or upholstered ones; shared hats and hair ornaments or sweaters and coats hanging side by side and touching. Young children tend to have lice more than older ones because they're in closer physical contact. They like hugs and they want to be right up on you. Some teachers discourage head-to- head contact in their classrooms in an effort to control lice.

Lice do not jump or fly, they just crawl. They do not care if hair is squeaky clean or needing to be washed. To take it a bit further, even though one of the worst cases of lice I ever saw was on biracial sisters, my observation has consistently been that head lice do not prefer my kind of kinky, black folks, natural, braided, or dread loc'd hair that we condition and maintain with gel and hair grease. They prefer naturally straight, what would be referred to as white people's type hair. This is why I had no problem whatsoever, searching through my white children's hair, commandeering the little creepy crawlers with my fingers, smashing them, and throwing them into the trash. Nothing a little handwashing won't take care of. After all, they are not a health hazard and they do not carry disease.

I have been called a bitch and worse because I contacted

parents to inform them of the lice in their child's hair. I have used my own money to shampoo a child's hair and pick nits because I knew the family could not afford it. In part, I wanted to experience washing heads and picking nits for myself so I could really relate to the parents' dilemma. Helpful or not, in a litigation crazed society, that was a risk on my part.

Sometimes, smothering the hair and the creepy crawlers in mayonnaise or other non-toxic, greasy substance, leaving it on for an hour, and then shampooing, helps. This method does not kill nits; only the live lice. It's also important to wash the sheets, blankets, and hats; spray the furniture upholstery, and treat again in about a week to kill the newly hatched lice. The lice shampoos do not necessarily kill the nits, just like greasy substances don't. That's why you get one of those "nit picking" combs included with the shampoo, and that's where the term comes from. The eggs or "nits" must be pulled or picked off. It's a nuisance.

I have by no means seen everything, but in my practice, I've observed way more African American boys with scalp ringworm for whatever reason, and I've seen it result in significant hair loss and follicle damage. I had no issue dealing with the lice because they are creatures that could be picked out and smashed. But with tinea capitis, or ringworm, I use extreme care. The oral medication for tinea capitus is serious. The last I checked, bloodwork to ensure the liver was not being damaged, was necessary during treatment.

## Boogers

You read that correctly; this is a story about boogers. Now boogers, or congealed nasal substance of a slimy matter, come from mucous, which is a useful and necessary body substance.

Mucous keeps membranes moist. Kleenex® and other facial tissues and handkerchiefs, were created to help us keep boogers under control in a clean and tidy manner.

One of the not-so-great issues with boogers is their presence can result in disgusting habits, and not just children have these habits. Adults pick, or even seriously dig up their noses with their bare fingers, too; some in public. The story that I'm about to share is funny. Well, kind of. The two students thought it was hilarious, while it made me think of the diabetic mud hike story, and blood-sucking leeches.

Sometimes, boogers' existence can be complicated when a student is prone to nosebleeds, and students who have spontaneous nosebleeds are relatively common. Oftentimes, they're due to weather changes or extremes. A fifth-grade boy was brought in by his "representative" classmate/friend because he was having a nosebleed during recess. (We'll talk more about "representatives" later!) It was one of those nosebleeds that was taking a while to stop. In addition to other tactics, one thing I do is to plug the nostril with a small piece of cotton so that it doesn't bleed all over the place.

After several attempts and 15 minutes of what we thought was no more bleeding, we figured it had finally stopped. Generally, when I remove the cotton ball, there might be a small amount of blood or a tiny clot. But upon removing that cotton ball plug, six-inch long, half inch in diameter rope of bloody mucous came trailing out, fully intact, looking like a red, slimy nightcrawler. All three of us yelled "EEEWWWWW" at the same time, as I hurriedly collected it in several tissues, so it did not soil his clothing! I know. Nasty!

Now, the good thing was, it was more mucous than blood,

meaning the nosebleed was about done. The not so cool thing was, it was one of the most disgusting sights I've seen in school, and I'm sure the guys thought so, too. But, being fifth-grade boys, they broke out into hysterical laughter. I did too, mainly laughing at them.

The student's nose stopped bleeding, he was good to go, and his parents were informed. The two of them left, still laughing hysterically, telling their friends how disgustingly funny it was. They were not in the least bit concerned about any of the pathophysiology of a nosebleed. And all I could think of was worms and leeches.

## Vision Screenings

Back in the day, all we had to screen pre-K and kindergarteners was the old-school vision box. It was that rectangular box with a light in it, and a screen with the symbols or letters. You plugged it into the wall and the screen would illuminate. We had objects we would use to cover one eye so we could determine the visual acuity of each eye separately. Now there are Spot Machine vision screeners. Still not always perfect with four- and five-year-old children but read on about old-school screening shenanigans.

If you've ever worked with children four and five years of age, you know they can be clueless. That's not an insult, it's for real. Some of them are very immature and have no idea what you want them to do, even when you tell them. It's not uncommon for them to have the attention span of a gnat, so the instructions you just gave them can go in one ear and out the other. They're easily distracted by other conversations, other children, the phone ringing, the bell ringing, wind, odors, you name it. They may not know their shapes. They may be busy trying to look at the inside of the object that's occluding their eye, which clearly is right up a half inch or less away from their eyeball. On some days, knowing I needed to do 25 or more screenings, was something that if I were a drinker, could require a strong drink before, during and afterwards.

The process involved our standing there next to the vision box, 10 feet away from the child, with a pointer. We would point to the shape and they were supposed to tell us what the shape was. For young children, we used a chart referred to as Lea Symbols. The symbols used were a circle, a house, a square and an apple. If it was early in the school year, or if the teacher felt that his or her students needed reinforcement, we would provide them with the symbols on individual square cards, for review beforehand. Towards the end of the school year, the children usually knew the shapes. But they could not always verbalize them. Here's an example.

"What is this shape, Ronnie?" Silence. "Do you know what this is?" More silence. Then "A ball!" OK, ball, circle, I'll take that as long as he calls all of them, balls.

"What's this one?" More silence, and now he's turning sideways looking at who knows what on the wall. "Over here, Ronnie. We're almost done, and I have a sticker for you when you get finished." "A heart!" OK, heart, apple- fine, whatever. Again, as long as he's consistent.

By this time, I was becoming distressed at the thought of even five more children, let alone 15. I'd been working for the district for too many years, and this right here was frustrating. I was thinking about being on a beach, at the gym, in bed, driving in rush hour traffic... Anywhere but trying to pull shapes out of four- and five-year-old brains.

Next object on the chart was a square. "What's this one, Ronnie?" Momentary silence, then with a huge grin, he yelled out something that sounded like "gurtangula!"

Now there was silence on my part, and I was staring at his smiling, pleased-looking little face thinking, what in the entire world are you saying? "What did you say this is?" "Gurtangula" he said a little more carefully, still proud of himself.

Bless his heart. He meant rectangle. Even though it was not a rectangle, I knew what he meant because I've been working around children for way too long, and I know how they think. As long as he called all the other squares "gurtangula," I was good. I just needed to get through the test with as few distractions as possible.

One more symbol to go. It was the house. Surely that won't be a problem, I thought. I pointed to it. "Roof" he yells! OMG, I thought to myself. I just want to be done with this! I guess he said that because I pointed close to the top of the house.

We got through the test. This is not a geometry lesson. This is again, to screen for visual acuity. So, ball, heart, roof, gurtangula- WHAT- EVER. He passed.

"Ronnie, did you know this shape is a square? Not a rectangle, a square. Can you say square?" He says square. "And this is a house. You did very well! Which sticker do you want?" He chose one and went away smiling, with his four-and-a-half-year-old self.

Wiping sweat off my brow, I went and got the next student. But I needed a drink, the beach, my bed, to be in rush hour traffic, something!

As an aside, I was prescribed eyeglasses as a fifth grader and have worn some kind of corrective lenses ever since. Many children get them younger. There are always those who are resistant to wearing them. All of my friends were nerdy, just like I was. We all wore eyeglasses, so it felt OK. But many are not on board with it. The child may be nerdy but would rather be "popular." The eyeglasses may be "ugly" or make the child feel ugly. Some children intentionally lose their glasses, as in, throw them away. Like into the neighbor's bushes three blocks away, or down the sewer. Like my little brother did with not one, but two pairs of eyeglasses.

And, you wonder why I sing.

## Eye Can See!

This next story was shared by one of my co-nurses.

"Third grader Crystal came skipping down the hall to catch me one day. She wanted to thank me for her new glasses. I sent a vision referral form home and Crystal's mother had taken her to an eye specialist. Crystal reported excitedly 'My mother didn't know I couldn't see until you sent the letter home.' She went on to elaborate 'I couldn't see which one was my house. Sometimes I listened for the gunshots and walked the other way. And, I could never understand how my sister could run through the house when my mother changed the furniture around. I had to walk slowly and get used to where everything was.'"

Can you imagine? I tried to envision myself in the child's position. Her situation reminded me of a home health story involving adults. An elderly Jewish couple lived in a luxury apartment building. Over their forty-plus year marriage, the husband had been a successful businessman, but according to his wife, he'd been rather mean.

Well, the husband lost his eyesight. Her way of getting back at him when she was angry was to rearrange the furniture and not tell him.

I told her that was not a good idea because it was a serious safety issue. When you get older, your reflexes are not as quick. Fall and injury hazard.

So, no. Sorry, just no.

## A Nine-by-Nine-Inch Box

During my last trip to Ibadan, Oyo State, Nigeria in West Africa, I made it a point to get permission to visit a school. It was a privately-run, church-supported elementary school. The focus of the school is learning and exceeding. There is no "mainstreaming" of special needs children. Those who have special needs (such as those who cannot eat on their own, who have a significant level of paralysis or whose brains do not function at a level where they can verbally communicate), are acknowledged as such and are provided for at a specialized facility. All parents are expected to have insurance for their children, which is very reasonable, and medication is not given at school. But then, there is not the level of pill dependency that we have here in the United States.

I do not believe there is necessarily anything wrong with having separate facilities based on individual and group needs, so long as the full focus is on the child's needs, and those needs are met. Different strokes for different folks. Some children excel in the arts, some science and some math. Some are good at public speaking; some are shy and do poorly reading out loud. Some are good at building and fixing things. There is absolutely nothing wrong with individualized attention, if it's equitable and specific to the student.

Parents should support their child in the role of a student, as much as possible. This means parents should be expected to act as parents and do everything within their power to provide for them, teach and expect appropriate behavior, see that they complete assignments, and cooperate with the school in the child's best interest. Part of parental support is holding the school accountable for the student's care, learning, and well-being while in school. It's a team effort, but the parent or legal guardian holds primary responsibility at all times.

Unfortunately, it's been my observation here in the United States, that in too many cases, parenting skills need addressing. Too many times, the school climate is not maximally conducive to learning, in part due to parental issues that have trickled down to their children. Without parental and school co-operation, there are problems.

Here are a couple of things I noticed while visiting a school in Ibadan. Even though it was an elementary school and the children were young and energetic, discipline problems were not tolerated. I could see some normal childhood mischief going on, and the teachers' responses were swift and no nonsense, but not harsh. Expectations were made clear with the students and the parents. Not one time did I see students disrespecting and talking back to adults, whether school personnel or parent. I did notice parents taking on the role and responsibility of being parents first, not their child's buddy or best friend. The culture is different. There were no "Bebe's kids" depicted as rowdy, loud, disrespectful children known to belong to the stereotypical Bebe in 'hood stories, and the parents did not defend their child with the suggestion that their baby could do no wrong. It was also understood that you were in a school, not a medical facility. No spending time in the nurse's office unnecessarily, and medical issues with children were expected to be addressed by the parents. As a matter of fact, there was no dispensary, and the medical supply consisted of a nine-inch by nine-inch metal box with a lid, that contained a couple of rolls of gauze, a few bandages, a tube of ointment, and a few safety pins. There were not several bottles of ADHD (attention deficit hyperactivity disorder) and ADD (attention deficit disorder) medications in a locked cabinet with other medicines, needing to be given out to make sure a student could make it through the day without becoming problematic to self or others. And if the child was on medication, the parents were expected to arrange to give it before, and then after school.

In my school nursing career, I'd say the overwhelming majority of parents have been supportive and diligent with their children's education process. But as the United States continues to suffer economically and even socially; as the gap between the haves and the have-nots widens; as more and more people find themselves in constant survival mode, the fallout is evidenced through our children. I think about children I mentioned earlier who I've seen at 8:30 or 9:00 a.m. with fevers of 101 or higher. Then out of five emergency phone numbers provided, none work. I consider the parents who are still in bed when their students leave home (the ones who the students say do not have jobs), as well as the children who arrive 30 to 45 minutes before school starts and stand outside before the school is open, even in the harshness of Cleveland winter weather. Then there are the ones who arrive an hour late on a regular basis. Or the second-grade student who tells me he was absent the day prior because his mother could not get out of the bed to get him ready and he was afraid to leave the house by himself. I do not know why these things happen, but they are not uncommon occurrences.

I'm not here to pass judgement. Instead, I feel compelled to share these observations because behind the scenes in the United States, we have some messiness going on, which could lead to potential crises. Having stayed with private families (with school-age children) three out of four of my visits to Ibadan, I can honestly say, having less is not always bad and having (or being fixated on accumulating) more, is not always good.

This is my question. Here in the United States there's a new campaign complete with T-shirts stating, "every school deserves (needs) a school nurse" or "every child deserves a school nurse." I have one of those shirts, and although it was not the case of every school needing a nurse on staff, oftentimes all day, every day; and although I didn't agree at first, I've started to agree over the last five years or so. Why is that? How did so many of our students and families get to the point of needing medical and other survival issues addressed, in school? Why are so many of our children on medication to control their behavior? Why are some so angry and violent? Why has juvenile diabetes risen so much? Why are our children suffering from childhood obesity? Why do so many come to school hungry or may not have dinner? These issues contribute to hours of learning time lost from being in the dispensary, seeing the nurse. I'm not referring to students with a diagnosis. I'm talking about the vague discomforts that really should be addressed at home. Why, with all of our resources, do we have such dysfunction? Do we realize we are quickly dropping down to the bottom of the ladder? Do we know if this keeps up, the next generation of adults will not be able to adequately care for themselves, let alone compete on an international level? Do we realize that their safety, security and well-being could seriously be compromised? What's going to happen to our next generation? Our children and grandchildren? How are other countries dealing with their children?

On my next visit to West Africa, my plan is to visit a public school, as well as a special needs facility for school-age children. And if I have another layover in Paris, I'd love to get permission to visit a school or two there as well. I'd like to see what "special needs" is defined as in other countries, and how those societies provide for the needs. But for now, I keep thinking about that very simple, nine-by-nine-inch box.

---

*Teenagers*

---

# Weaves, Fingernails, Ridiculousness and Tragedies

Most of my nursing experiences in schools have come from elementary school assignments, but there were several years where I was full time at high schools, covering ninth through twelfth grades. Several of these next memories are from the same school. On my first day at one assignment, I found the school's principal was the assistant principal from when I was in high school! Such a pleasant surprise and one of the perks of working in the same school district I attended growing up! We recognized each other immediately, even though many years had passed. As a student, occasionally I would forget my eyeglasses at home, and request an out-of-the-building pass to go home and get them. While at home, I'd make myself a sandwich before going promptly back to school. I could only go if it was study hall period, and I had to be back before a class. That was back in the day when students could be out during the day and not be in danger; when there were still stay-at-home, neighborhood moms watching out; when there were working dads in two-parent households; and when most of us would not push our parents' limit by doing something totally unacceptable that would have our parents go straight off on us.

Here are a few things I experienced with older children.

## When You Have to be Flyy

High school girls can be very concerned about their appearance. This means fingernails. Oh, and hair weaves and nose rings. As an aside, I didn't know white girls wear fake hair/extensions, too. That is until I was getting makeup done for a photo shoot once. The lady in the chair across the room from me was some kind of way, having extension hair fused onto her own hair with a flat iron. Who knew? Certainly not me.

I've had girls ask me to remove nail tips that have been on for months, making it such that they are hanging on to the tip of the nail, causing splits close to the nailbed. "Miss, can you get this off?" Oh, good grief, I think to myself. Does your mother know it's hanging like that? Sometimes I can get them off, sometimes I call home because it's too much of a risk. Then there are the weaves that have not been well maintained, and have been in way too long, until they're at the point of damaging the girl's natural hair and scalp. In our 'hoods, it's called edges.

Once a student came in frantic, saying how glad she was I was the nurse that day. She had just gotten her nose pierced the night before, and she knew my nose was pierced. If any of you have a nose piercing, you know how long it takes for it to heal to the point where you can leave the stud or ring out for any length of time. It can take as long as a year, maybe more, or else you run the risk of it quickly closing up. If you get yours pierced, you really should be clear in asking the person who pierces it, if they are professional, about the healing process. I also think it should be a professional. I learned through trial and error. Unfortunately, she had forgotten it was pierced, wiped her nose, and knocked the stud out. Fortunately, or unfortunately, I remembered doing that, too.

We got it back in, but it was not easy. She was more worried about being cute than the inconvenience and discomfort of putting it back in. I told her if she knocked it out again, I was going to just take her entire nose off, so she would not have to worry about it. She gave me a hug and left with a little bit of a sore nose. She was cute, though!

## Thug Behavior

Periodically, fights would break out and I would be called to come and check for injuries, or the students would be sent to the dispensary. First thing one morning, a fight broke out. A young male student came to my office with a gash on his forehead. Because of my SICU training, dressings were a specialty of mine. This boy's cut was just a bit deeper than superficial, but was clean and relatively short, without a whole lot of bleeding. Nothing that cleaning and a couple of Steri-Strips couldn't handle.

This was back in the day of pagers. I had my school-issued pager sitting on the desk as I was attending to this child. You already know where I'm going with this. While I was fixing up his cut so he wouldn't have to take his ignorant self to the ER and get stitches (and might I say, I did a very good job), I'm convinced he stole my pager. I never did find it.

To top that off, his mother had the audacity to suck her teeth at me because I called and asked her, at the principal's request, to come to the school to get her son. She was still asleep. So what, I thought. Get up, he's your son. Needless to say, I wanted to drop-kick both of them.

## In-School Tragedy

While I do my best to encourage students to stay in school, I also listen to what I call the Voice. The Voice provides me with intuitive messages. Intuition and nursing do not necessarily go hand in hand. And certainly, it should not be used as a primary source of reference. If that were the case, anyone could be designated as a medical provider. Still, the Voice can be quite useful.

Again, as a parent first, nurse second, I address my students' issues as I would address my own sons', as much as possible. Sometimes I give them firm pushback on their agendas, and sometimes I give in. One day, a young lady came to the dispensary asking if she could call her mother to get permission to go home because she wasn't feeling well. I don't remember her being what I would call sick, but she was not a Frequent Flyer, and the Voice was strongly urging me to call her mother so she could go.

When her mom arrived, they gave each other a hug and mom asked me if her daughter could wait with me while she took care of some brief business in the main office. Five to 10 minutes later, I got a phone call asking me to come to the office immediately. Fortunately, I was able to lock up the main part of the dispensary and leave the student in the outer office waiting area.

When I got to the front office, her mother was on the floor, breathing, but unconscious. After looking at her blown (largely dilated) pupils, I told the principal and the secretary to call EMS immediately because it did not look good.

Long story short, the mother was taken to the hospital and auntie came to pick up the student. Mom was in the hospital about a week and died of a massive stroke. I couldn't believe it. To this day, I wonder what would have happened if I had encouraged the student to stay in school and had not called her mother. Would the student have gone home and found her mother dead?

When her daughter returned to school two weeks later, she came in and we hugged each other. She was crying and wondering why her mother had to die, especially like that. All I could offer was, in an odd way, perhaps the student's feeling a bit under the weather had been good. Perhaps it was God's way of making sure she and her mother had a chance to see and hug each other while her mom was fully conscious and looked well, before she died.

Her daughter thought about it and as painful as it still was, was comforted by it.

## Out-of-School Tragedy

Through all the dysfunction and drama, I've worked with a lot of very good kids with attentive parents who are for the most part, on top of things. There was a student whose mother I ended up befriending. She did an awesome job of braiding hair, so I would go to her to get mine done. This went on nicely for close to a year. Then one day I got a call from a school administrator who told me the boy had been on his bike and another teen had intentionally hit him with the car he was driving, killing him. There were other boys in the car, too.

That incident and the parent having the stroke in the front office were two of the worst memories I have of school nursing. I wonder where the boy who hit him is today and I wonder where the passengers who were in the car are, and what they thought at the time of the incident. Although I checked up on the student's mother a few times after that, she ended up moving out of town and we lost contact. All of it was too much for her. I still think about them. He was a very gentle-spirited, intelligent young man. I think the driver was just probably being hormonal, playing around and didn't intend to kill him. But that's what happened and there was no turning back. Like some kids say, "they play too much."

## $125 Not-So-Joyful Ride

Not only are some of my high school students amazingly naive, they also think we as adults were never young and we should trust and believe whatever they say. I avoid sending students home walking during the day whenever I can. But sometimes, after calling the parents, I'm requested to let the student walk home. Mom or dad could be at work unable to leave, there may not be a car in the family, it may not be running or there may not be anyone else available to come for the student. But I never let them dial the number. I look up the number myself, dial it, ask who I'm speaking to, tell them the general issue, let the student speak, then ask to speak to the parent/guardian again before the call is ended. As an aside, there've been times when I've had to take the phone, apologize to the parent, hang up, and send the angry student to the principal or back to class. I don't tolerate the way some of these students speak to their parents when they can't get their way. Talk to your mom, dad, gramma or whomever, out of my office if you must speak to them with downright disrespect.

So, a young lady came in whining about going home. I had never seen her before; thus, she was not categorized as a Frequent Flyer. Because of this, I gave her the benefit of the doubt and wrote her an out-of-the-building pass after getting the OK from her mother. The following week, I found out the student had headed to her boyfriend's house instead, lost the out-of-the-building pass I had given her, and because she didn't have a pass, was picked up by the police for being truant. Her mother was assessed a $125 fine.

You may wonder how as a sub, I get to know who's a Frequent Flyer, and who is not. Well, sometimes you can tell by the Post-it® notes of phone numbers the full-time nurse may have on the office wall or attached to the computer. Or by the daily log of charting. Or, because I'm regularly called to certain schools, I get to know the students. Some students' names are committed to memory on the first day because of their behaviors, bad or good.

Speaking of documentation, we are required to keep duplicate copies of any out-of-the-building passes we write. This is important if, God forbid, anything was to happen to a student, or if they came up missing. Girlfriend never came back to the dispensary, at least not while I was there. Probably in part because she was embarrassed and knew that I knew she had lied. I told one of her besties that when she saw her, to tell her I said her game was raggedy, she cost her mother a chunk of change, that I'd never write her an out-of-the-building pass again because she's not to be trusted, and that I really didn't want to see her in the dispensary unless she was shot or stabbed.

All exaggerations, but still. Older brats.

## Haints Be Gone

My mother used to talk about haints. Haints are said to be spirits that older people, especially African Americans to my knowledge, called ghosts, "vexed" or wayward spirits. My priesthood in the traditionalist practice of Ifa has exposed me to the very real issue of spiritual activity. Some of that activity is good and what I'd say is productive, some is kind of bothersome.

As a result of my trips to West Africa and Cuba, I regularly observe issues my elders talk to me about, in some of my students. These issues can be a challenge to validate medically, but it does not negate the fact that I still see it. The issues are emotional, psychological and spiritual. If you've ever gone into a room, house or other environment, and it just didn't feel right, you know what I'm talking about.

Except on rare occasions, I never left school for lunch break, especially with the presence of diabetic students and other "stuff" constantly going on. I prepared my lunch at home and grazed off and on as I got a chance. One of my larger dispensaries had four separate rooms. I used to let students lie down on occasion in one of the smaller inner rooms. It was where I would occasionally go as well to get a 15-minute power nap on what was designated as my lunch hour. Never did I fall fully asleep. I'd just shut down and relax my mind. It was enough to refresh me for the afternoon.

Then came the day when I could not get up off the cot. It felt as though a sticky net had been tossed over me and was holding me down. Try as I might, I could not get myself up. I was plenty conscious enough to feel what was going on, but for the life of me, I could not shift out of that "dimension." I remember thinking to myself that I was going to be trapped up in there and the custodian or cleaner would come after school had closed, and find me in there, wilding out.

Finally, I struggled my way off the cot and out of that dimension, sweating and breathing hard. I ran into the outer, main room wondering "What in the heck was THAT?" I brushed myself off, got some water, and decided I would never lie down back there again.

Meanwhile, I told my mother about the experience. She grew up on a farm in North Carolina. "Haints," she said. "Sounds like haints."

Well, I'll tell you what. School building or not, the next day, I brought in charcoal for burning incense, camphor, frankincense, myrrh, copal- whatever I had at home, and smoked the joint out before school started. The crazy energy that had accumulated in there, had to go. This was years ago before asthma and other allergies started manifesting in children in record numbers.

The kids came in talking about "What's that smell, Miss? It's kind of weird." "No weirder than what it's getting rid of" I told them. "And while you're over there, open that window please."

# 5 SAY THAT

This is another section dedicated to children. Kids will say some of anything. Their discretion filter has not developed yet. Most of the things they say are amusing, but a lot is not. Like the first grader who came into my office to say, "my mom told me not to talk about we have bedbugs." Cleary the bedbugs were bothering her. This section is dedicated to a few of the things I've heard over the years, some of which was out of line. Remember: this is 'hood medical, so some of what you hear is going to be just that. 'Hood.

---

*Young Children*

---

"My gramma phone cut off," said the nine-year-old child who came in within 10 minutes of school starting, stating his stomach hurt. He said it just like that, poor grammar and all. So, while dude is laid out sideways on the cot, head propped up on his arm looking like a little old man, he proceeded to tell his family's business. "All they phones is cut off. All dem gotta get they money together and pay to get 'em cut back on." ("Lil bruh" I was thinking, "your grammar in this school setting is horrible. Do you talk like that in class?") The child was listening in on and adding his comments to everything going on in the dispensary. But when he started talking about his mother's boyfriend and the old car he needed to get rid of, it was RTC for him. "Here's your pass, you can return to class," at which time he hopped off the cot, adjusted his shirt, and strolled out. Literally strolled out.

\*

I try to give good examples of healthy lifestyles, so sometimes I tell my students I go to the gym. A second-grade boy wanted to know what I do at the gym. I told him I lift weights, walk or run the treadmill, sometimes jump rope. It was at that point he stopped me and told me adults should not jump rope. "Why not?" I wanted to know. "Because y'all are too old and big and you might fall and break something." Boy bye. You RTC, too.

\*

"Miss, why is one of your eyes darker than the other?" "Huh? What do you mean? My eyeball?" "No. What's that purple stuff called? That purple stuff right there." The eight-year-old girl comes up and almost touches my left eyelid. (\*Sigh\* That's not purple. It's Midnight Burgundy eye shadow, little girl.) See? This is why it's important to be very mindful of what you have on and how you present yourself. Once children decide they have a relationship with you where they can easily talk to you, they'll be asking you all sorts of things, as well as voicing their opinions, including monitoring your makeup, clothing and any little flaws, and remembering it for future reference, good or not so good. It's part of their learning process.

*

Speaking of makeup and things, I had a photo shoot scheduled right after school one day and needed to wear my hair hat—sorry, I mean wig, to cover my locs. I was told not to wear any makeup, as the makeup artist was going to do it for me once I arrived. Even though I wear very little makeup daily, I "needed" that eyebrow enhancer, and mascara. My children notice and comment about everything, even when the purple eye shadow is uneven! I couldn't imagine what gems would come out of their little mouths regarding a straight-hair, bob-cut wig and my undone eyebrows!

Especially that wig! I've worn locs for 20 years. Even I had to get used to looking at myself in a wig! It would have been more time efficient for me to just wear the wig to school, but, if I had gone in there that morning like that, they would have been totally confused, staring at me, asking a million questions as to why and what, thinking about it and would have been right up on me examining every detail, wanting to touch it, shamelessly and matter-of-factly voicing their very honest and blunt opinions. Some of the preschoolers might not have even recognized me. Some might even have been afraid of me! I know of younger children who've been afraid of people or otherwise "disrupted" for a variety of appearance-related reasons.

Nope. I couldn't do it. I was admittedly being a chicken-shit. Instead, when I got to the shoot location, I sat in the parking lot in the car, and while waiting for the previous client to finish, I slowly pinned up my hair, and took off the brow and lash makeup with some lotion, effectively destroying the one contact lens I wear in my mono-visioned right eye. Good thing I carry a pair of eyeglasses in the car so I could see to drive home.

I got inside to my shoot on time, and all went well, thank goodness. I was in a three-month assignment at that school, and those children were used to me. They would have been on it for the next week, looking at me crazy and asking all sortsa questions. No. Just, no.

So, let me introduce myself again. "My name is Nurse Barbara, I'm a coward and I can't with those chilrens because I've worked with them for too long. I know them."

The power of children!

*

Back to nose rings. This time, kindergarteners. The Three Amigas. One of them came in daily for her inhaler. Then another one started coming with her. The next day a third one came, too. All of them had some vague and minor complaint, while smiling. I think they just wanted to leave the classroom because they were bored. One of them who was admiring my nose ring, said "I like your that." "My that? You mean, this?" I asked her as I pointed to the tiny, sparkly stud I had in that day. "Yes," she said. I told her it was a nose ring. She and her friends were right up on me as I sat there, staring at my nose. The stud was very tiny. "My mom has a nose ring," one of them said. "Mine doesn't," said one of the others. "She just has pimples." See why I can't with them? See?

Sometimes my kids try to play jokes on me. For the most part, I know who to trust and who not to, so I let them. Lil dude comes in one morning and offers me a Jelly Belly®. I had no idea I was about to be BeanBoozled. "Pick one…" he said. I picked one and it was Dog Food flavor, much to my chagrin. OK, funny, I could hang! He showed me the box and I saw there were flavors like Barf, Lawn Clippings, Booger and Stinky Socks. (Who thought those up?) Then he said, "I know some adult flavors, too. My dad told me." Uh oh, here we go, I thought to myself. He leaned over and whispered in my ear, "Pole Stripper." Dude! Goodbye!

*

There are also quite a few shy students. They come in and look at me and if I ask them what's wrong, they stare at me and say nothing. Or whisper inaudibly. Or just hand me the paper from the teacher. Many times, children with shy personalities are accompanied to the dispensary by a spokesperson, or who I like to call their representative. Remember the Booger story? Good example.

A second-grade girl with large blue eyes, came in and was looking at me like she had no idea what to say when I asked her what was wrong. Her representative was matter of fact, vocal, with trendy eyeglasses. "She needs her temperature taken to see if she's sick" said the representative. "Alrighty then," I said as I got the thermometer out. "Well, no fever," I told the client and her representative when I got finished. "Did you have breakfast?" Blank stare. "She wants to know if you had breakfast" said the representative to her client. She shook her head no. I gave her a snack. When she was done, I asked the client if she felt better and she shook her head yes, smiling. Then I thanked the representative. Her response was "We have the same last name, that's why we're friends. But, we're not 'delated.'" I simply smiled and nodded, as they left out hand in hand. I could have corrected her and told her that she meant 'related'. But I chose not to. She's smart. She'll figure it out in due time.

Kudos to teachers for knowing their students, including who needs "representation" even if only for a few months. #futurelawyers #patientadvocates

\*

While this is not medical, I find it fascinating and absolutely wonderful, the number of young children who are bilingual, some as young as kindergarten. They translate for me, their parents, and some of their friends and family members. Most of them have immigrated to the U.S. from places like Asia, Puerto Rico, South America, and various African nations. There are two schools in Cleveland where most new immigrants begin their U.S. education. I always tell them how wonderful it is to be bilingual and encourage them to continue to study. There are numerous jobs waiting for them if they can speak more than one language fluently. #winning

\*

There are quite a few students who receive medication for ADHD (attention deficit hyperactivity disorder), ADD (attention deficit disorder), and others. I think in part, this could be due to a breakdown in family structure, routine, discipline, food additives and more, in addition to inherited tendencies. For several reasons, some good and some not so good, many receive their medication during school hours. Truth be told, some students won't take their medication from their parents.

Before I go further, "*won't*" take their medication from their parents? I've had several parents over the years say this. I do not understand because there were very few if any things my sons didn't do that I asked or told them to do, short of hang up their coats or something. Perhaps refusal to comply with the parental figure is a part of the dysfunction, but I still do not understand a child "refusing" to do what they're told in a matter such as this. However, remember when I said sometimes children will take suggestions from someone who's not a parent, if they know and trust them? This is important to remember.

Many meds can be put in food as a creative and discreet way of giving it. We require many children to have a mouth check after they're given their pill, to make sure they swallowed it. In all fairness, some older children say they do not like the way they feel after taking their medication. While this may be legitimate, there still needs to be cooperation between parent and child, with physician input if problems persist. But the reality is, oftentimes the school nurse or other designated staff member, is responsible.

Two fifth-grade boys came into the dispensary. The taller, athletically built child with a gregarious personality, introduced himself and told me he was there to take his medication. His representative was a much smaller, wiry boy with what would be considered nerdy glasses. "I have to bring him down here to take his medicine," he said, referring to his gregarious, bigger client/friend. "He's crazy."

Whoa! That was extremely blunt, and I wasn't prepared for it at all, but I said nothing. The client was pleasant, looking at me matter-of-factly like, "hey, it is what it is." He took his medicine, said thank you and goodbye, and they left.

I could spend all day "correcting" children's perspectives on things. Once again, I chose to observe. These two had a relationship and understanding of what was going on, what was necessary, and why. I was an outside observer, new to their world.

Some days in situations such as this, I don't know if according to their world, I'm correct or incorrect. Especially being a substitute nurse. Most times, I'd rather them feel comfortable enough with me to say what they're feeling, versus them not saying anything because it may be incorrect.

Other days, I just don't know, and when I don't know, I lean towards observing and keeping my opinions or corrections to myself.

*

Sixth-grade boy: "Miss (while pointing at a fresh, lightly bleeding cut on his arm), can I borrow a Band-Aid®?" Me: "So, let me make sure I understand you. You want me to lend you a Band-Aid® so you can put it on your arm on that bleeding cut, and then you wanna give it back? Naw..." Both of us laughed while I had him clean it off and dress it. "You give out bandages for dressings, not lend them out. We do not want that contaminated stuff back" I told him. We laughed again; he got it. I know what he meant, but this was a teachable moment on correct word usage and comprehension, in addition to my being able to make sure he knew how to take care of a minor first aid issue. Sometimes the situation presents itself as such.

*

Rant from a Frequent Flyer kindergartener waiting for her parents coming to get her: "When I was little I threw up and they gave me crackers and flowers when I was five I had a toy box are you going to give me a whoopin on my birthday? I get a whoopin on my birthday but are those cameras?" (Me: Where?) "Those." (Me: No, they're lights) "Well how can you see someone without a camera?" (Me: Huh?) "Where's the dog? (FYI, the dog she was referring to was one of two mascot dogs at that small, non-public school.) "I had a dog, but it ran away so we had to throw out the dog food so mice wouldn't get it and so it wouldn't get bad like sometimes the bread gets if we don't eat it fast enough and I don't like bread all the time only sometimes." Aside from the specific questions, do you see how these sentences all run together with just enough punctuation for you to know if sentences were questions or statements? I wrote it like this because it's exactly how she was talking to me. It was mind boggling to say the least. (Unfortunately, it reminded me of how some young adults post on social media.) Then she started singing a song. She vomited twice, but in between those times, she was singing or talking non-stop in continuous, run-together sentences, and otherwise bouncing off the walls. Dad came to get her. He said she never throws up at home. He also said mom does the same thing. Not the throwing up part. The incessant talking in run-together sentences.

Poor dad.

*

Over my adult life, I recall a few dreams where I met people in a dream before I've met them in person. A couple of days before I started a month-long assignment, I dreamed of a boy and a girl. I saw them very clearly. I did not know them, but when I got to the school, I met them. They looked just like in the dream. One was diabetic, one was the representative. The representative had been taught so well by the regular nurse she came pretty close to knowing the correct dosages for his insulin. She knew when the number meant the client needed insulin, when he needed water, when he needed a snack, when he needed an adjustment for gym– She was on point. I asked her if she was going to be a nurse and she told me no, an artist. A girl after my own heart! I told her she could do both. Like me. And they both were first graders.

*

Over the last couple of years, I've been building my brand. One way of brand building is through social media. Even my elementary students are up on the latest social media trends. One day while trying to eat and add a picture and commentary to my Instagram profile, one of my busy-body, eight-year-old boys came in and was all over my shoulder looking at my profile picture. It was a picture taken during a photoshoot for my CD, a headshot that might be considered a glamour shot, hair done, professional makeup, you know the deal. The child proceeds to say, "Aw, Nurse Barbara, that picture is raw! But you don't look like that today." (Me side-eyeing him.) For anyone who doesn't know, "raw" can mean: hottt, slaying, fly, fabulous, gorgeous, awesome – like that. But the child made sure to tell me I was not representing all like that on a daily basis. This right here! This is another reason why I did not wear that wig with no makeup to school!

*

"My leg itches." "Why?" "Because I got bit. It was a tarantula under my bed, then I saw it on my sister's bed." (A tarantula? Seriously? Another blank stare moment) I gave her some cold water in a glove, to put on it. To this child, a large spider probably did look like a tarantula.

I can relate. As a child, I was terrified of spiders. While in Cuba some years back to present at a conference, they were loose, roaming freely in nature. The good thing is the one I saw was pretty slow. (I still stuffed a rolled-up towel under the door gap of our hotel room.)

Then there was the huge spider in my bathroom sink one night. I usually don't turn on the light, but this time I wanted to make sure that the water wasn't dripping, and there it was. Luckily, it had been doused with water, so it was slow. I doused it with more, got some tissue, and smooshed it in my hands, all in about five seconds. Or the furry jumping spider who decided it was a good idea to be in my bathtub with me. I was determined it would not use me as an island of temporary respite from the hot water I sit in after my workouts. Between me tryna scoop it out in my hands full of water, and finally resorting to hitting it with the bath brush, Spidey met its demise.

In my mind, either I was going to get it or risk it getting on me. It could not win. I've come a long way with spiders, because I didn't hurt myself trying to get away from it.

*

Then there was my friend's son. We weren't even at school. We were at my sister's house having a social gathering. This ten-year-old heard me saying I was a school nurse and said "Eewww!" "WHAT?" I asked. The child told me he had a "bad experience" with the school nurse because she would talk too close to his face, she had dentures and the dentures would make clicking noises when she talked. (Blank staring at this child, too) "And" he continued, "she had bad breath."

I was speechless. What do you say to that?

\*

An ADHD student who loved to color, came in to show me a picture of a frog he had colored. The picture had a Puerto Rican flag in the background. The flag was brightly colored as was the frog. "Do you think Puerto Rican frogs just say 'ribbit' or do they say it in Puerto Rican?" I was caught way off guard on this one. "Um… I don't really know!" He left the picture for me declaring "I think they just say regular ribbit." Alrighty then!

\*

Then there was Christmas. I wear either an elf hat, antlers or other types of amusing and decorative head gear. The kids like it and it adds to the festive atmosphere of the season. So, one day as I was walking down the hall with antlers on, the preschoolers were on their way to the gym in their nice little line. "Oooooo, children," their teacher said. "What do you see? Look at her head? What animal is that?" One by one they started saying "Reindeer!" That is until this one child out of the clear blue says, "Donkey!" The teacher was horrified. I immediately busted out laughing because essentially, I had been called an ass by a child! LOL

\*

Please pardon the language you're about to see. I do not use foul language much in my everyday life. I especially don't with children. That's a no-no, even though I've been called Bs, Hs, etc. But, part of my relationship with children has to do with being able to meet them halfway and understand some of how they think and talk, and why. So, consider the third-grade child who had to be in the dispensary for his medication/treatment daily. The child was precocious to say the least, manipulative, somewhat stubborn, but still very likeable, sometimes funny, and very smart. "Nurse Barbara, you always be talmbout 'hold on, gimme a minute'... – I can just get those batteries myself." The batteries he was "talmbout" were on the top shelf of my cupboard above the sink, about a foot away from the ceiling. Me: "Hold up, I'mabouta get 'em in a minute." Child: "I can get 'em, you takin too long." Me: "I said wait, lemme finish with Sarah." Dude proceeds to climb up on the sink counter with his shoes on, so he could reach the top cupboard, *anyhow*.

At this point, he became one of the sons I gave birth to. I immediately cleared Karen and her representative out of the dispensary, shut the door, and went straight in, telling OG (original gangster) Wannabe, "Get your ass offa my sink top, before I kick it. I told you wait, and that's what I meant. I'm the OG (old girl) as in, your elder who's old enough to be your gramma, and I'm the authority figure up in this joint. You will do as I ask." The look on his face as he silently climbed down, all the while not taking his eyes offa me, was priceless. I'd had enough and was not bustin' a smile because wasn't nothing funny. I finished his treatment in silence and sent his hard-headed self on to class. The next day, all was normal, I greeted him with the usual smile and fist-bump as he said with amazement in his voice, "Nurse Barbara, you said a swear word to me yesterday!" We then had a discussion about the importance of following directions from authority figures and using good judgement in the first place. I reminded him that his mother and I had a conversation the first day of school when she came in to meet me, where she basically acknowledged his "playful," silly, and yes, hard-headed nature, and told me to feel free to handle it. "I would not hit you, and I would not curse you out. But you understood and came down after I said that, didn't you? Be glad I didn't call your mother and tell her, else she'd have gone in on you again, once you got home." On rare occasions, and under certain circumstances, we may feel the need to go there. This was one of those times. But we can't be stupid about it. He and I had a rapport prior to that incident, and we had no more problems afterwards, even though his personality remained the same. Limits are crucial for our children. Teachable moments of the 'hood kind. #BlackLivesMatter

*

Once a student came in whose dad worked as a security guard in a neighboring school. She swears he told her a student's book bag went through the metal detector with a live cat in it that was undetected, after which the child let the cat loose in the classroom. Says the child got the cat out of a tree on her way to school and put it in her book bag.

OK, come on now. Really, lil girl?

## Teenagers

I don't like donuts all like that. Well, mostly I don't need them. But sometimes in my attempt not to be extreme about my fitness journey, and to remember what gooey, sugary stuff tastes like, I indulge, especially when they're sitting out on the table in the staff lounge, free for the taking. So, as I came out into the hallway, a tall dude was walking by and immediately started walking right up on me, step by step. I have to refer to him as tall dude because he was at least 6'2"; a thin, somewhat pale white child. He had already been to see me that morning for a heat pack to put on his leg that was cramping from basketball the day before. The heat pack was my signature bootleg joint, made out of a glove filled with warm water. They're cheap and effective. "Aww, see Miss? Lemme get a donut!" Here we go, I thought to myself. He is not going to go away easily. "Aww, see? They're not mine and they're for the staff," I replied. "C'mon Miss, get me a donut, PLEASE." "They're not mine, son..." By this time, he was literally right up on me, all 135 pounds or so of his narrow, 15-year-old self, eyeing the donut which I had already taken one bite out of. He was going nowhere. "HERE, TAKE HALF, JUST BACK UP OFFA ME, JEEZ!" I said this half smiling and half mean-mugging, as I broke off half and gave it to him. You should've seen him smiling, happy to get that half of a donut, as he walked down the hall ignoring his friends who were asking him where he got it from. The majority of kids are cool and really do like and respect the adults who work with them. They appreciate limits but will push them on occasion. This interaction was harmless. He was not diabetic, and he was narrow as a rail. His weight had not caught up with his height. They like attention and they like to sometimes be your friend. And sometimes you let them win.

Especially when you don't need donuts.

*

But then, sometimes students are horribly disrespectful. And some of them only understand "ghettoese." You know, like Chinese, Maltese or Senegalese? Once again, pardon the language. This story is from a coworker. A high school boy called her an old, stupid bitch. Her immediate come-back, straight-faced as what: "Yo' momma." Silence. He was stunned. Then he smiled ever so slightly and apologized. "My bad, Miss."

I hope none of you are ever called a bitch, especially by anyone significantly younger. It's a terrible feeling of disbelief, frustration, disrespect, anger and of desired "smack-tivity" as in, I'd like to turn into some really old-school parent or grandparent.

I've been called disrespectfully out of my name by a student or two. A couple of parents also. It's not a good feeling. It's especially bothersome when you don't even know the person, or all you've ever done was try to help. This, however, can be real in our communities, but thankfully is not the norm.

*

Or, how about being told by a high school student in one of the impromptu, unsolicited group hangouts in the dispensary, "Yeah, my daddy was a pimp and he had 'hos." OK, it's going to be one of those conversations this time. I believe a lot of what these kids say. What would be the point of lying or creating stories such as this? A lot of times, talking about their lives is cathartic. Especially if the listening ear does just that: listens and passes no judgement or opinion, unless it's a seriously debatable topic. Sometimes I'd allow older students to come in on their lunch break or study hall. I was kinda glad they felt like I hosted a safe space where they could talk and keep it "100" like they say these days.

With the whole idea of a 'ho ('hood for whore) in mind, here's an example of 'hood language seriously misunderstood or misinterpreted. It came from a movie where there was a clear satire on cultural perspectives and differences. A kind-hearted, but much older white woman was principal of a high school that seemed to be of mixed ethnicities, but still had clear 'hood elements. Remember, 'hood perspectives and behaviors can be across ethnic and racial lines. Some of the most 'hood young men I've encountered were white, and it's not necessarily because they affiliated with black children. If you have 'hood mentality or it's in your DNA, you just do. Don't ask me how or why, it just is. And, I ain't mad at 'em, as they say, because some of them are the kindest individuals you'd ever wanna meet. The principal was clearly limited in her knowledge of popular language, but despite her cultural limitations, as principal, she still had to be vocal and exert a level of authority.

One of her lines, after chastising a couple of students for fighting, was (paraphrased), "I just don't know why James would call Anthony's mother a garden tool!"

Say what? I busted out laughing while it clearly went over the heads of many people in the theater. James insulted Anthony and his mother by calling her a 'ho, as in a loose woman, not a hoe as in a garden tool. LOL! Who *wrote* that line?

*

This observation is not really about something someone said, it's about social media. Having a social media presence has been beneficial and quite informative. In addition to building my brand and promoting business-related activities, I can keep up with trends and out-of-town family members. However, certain platforms are losing their youthful users. When I ask some of my students, or even my sons and nephews why, they give me answers like "people are crazy," "they play too much," "they be doing too much" or "it's too many old people on there." It can also be looked at as promoting all things "fake." What you see with filters online is not necessarily what you get in person.

And, speaking of "ole pipo" (it originally took me a minute to realize this was another way of saying "old people") IMHO (in my humble opinion), people my age and older do not need to have our pictures enhanced with filters that give us cat and dog ears, snouts and whiskers. Although I'm not close to her age, a 75-year-old lady asked me if I knew how to get on one of those platforms. I told her, "We don't. We're too old for that!" It seems social media is used a lot by lonely people of any age. It fosters a sense of connection. But at some point, we have to draw the line. Then there's YouTube. YouTube provided a bit of a link between a high school student and me, when he was feeling like not participating. First thing in the morning, he came to the dispensary with some vague complaint, no fever, no other symptoms, and was mumbling. I absolutely hate when they intentionally won't speak up. "I'm sorry, what did you say your name is?" "Mumble-uh-bub" it sounded like he was saying, barely moving his mouth. After the second time, I was becoming annoyed. Yes, he could have written it down, but remember. As a former critical care nurse, I listen to and pay attention to all potential signs and symptoms. Plus, it was the beginning of the school day. We hadn't been there an hour. "Please speak a little louder and clearer." Then it sounded like he was saying Malik. But, surely this reddish-blonde haired, fair-skinned white child was not named Malik! That made no sense. So, the child spells out "B-L-A-K-E" "Oh!" I said loudly with a big, goofy smile! "Like buh-LAH-kay on The Substitute!" The child started smiling and said in a quiet but normal tone of voice, "My nick name is buh-LAH-kay. My sisters call me that." We both laughed and he decided to go on to class "cured" and smiling.

Sometimes laughter is the only medicine.

*

High school girls are not only concerned about their appearances, but also the appearances of their parents or caregivers when they come to school. *PLEASE* parents, especially mothers and grandmothers, be mindful of that. It's embarrassing if you come with too tight or sheer leggings on, showing everything; with too much cleavage showing; your hair a hot mess, 'do rags, bonnets, pajamas, etc., because if you do, trust me, I'll hear conversations like "Jackie's momma came up here with those see-through leggings on. She too old for that. Jackie be so embarrassed."

Some of them talk about people's parents so badly, it makes me go immediately to the mirror to check myself and see what I'm looking like. I'd hate to be the topic of negative conversation. At that point they'd stop viewing me as a role model and no longer confide in me because they'd be talking about me.

*

Finally, there was a 17-year-old student who came to see me because he had a sore throat and a slight fever. When I asked if I should call his mother, he asked me to call his grandmother. Gramma made it clear that she was not available. Then he told me I'd have to call his case worker because he was living in a group home for boys. He was very honest about his mother having put him out, not wanting him to return home because he continued to smoke weed in the house when she asked him not to. Gramma just didn't want to be bothered. I felt bad for him because I could see the remorse in his face. It made me think about my own sons and nephews and what would happen if they were in a similar situation. Children make mistakes and can be hard-headed. Adults, too. Some do not learn until after they go to the proverbial "school of hard knocks" and are well into their adulthood. The good thing was, he was not on harder drugs, or on the streets, homeless. He also seemed to be honest about his responsibility in the mess. He said as long as he graduated from high school, maintained good behavior, found a job and or enrolled in school, the county would assist him in finding housing. He knew he was on his own and had to make it. Still, a part of me wished he was doing teenage things like playing sports and being active in after-school, extracurricular activities, hanging out with friends, etc. Ah, the choices we make.

Cause and effect.

# 6 HERE'S WHAT'S UP: A NURSING ASSESSMENT

## Self-Assessment and Transparency

Nursing as with really any job, occupation, work, or other venture, is usually selected based not only on a need for income, but also on personality traits, things we like, personal limitations and other considerations. Over time, we would be wise to reassess ourselves and consider changes that may need to be made. For many people, a constant, long-term routine is exactly what's wanted. I knew ladies who graduated from nursing school with me and started their careers in certain areas in the same hospital we graduated from, who were still in the same position 15 years later. That's a wonderful thing because I would think under those circumstances, they were really experts in their field. I, however, would have gone nuts. Change, variety and being motivated to learn something different are really important to me. The key is, we have to know ourselves. We have to also know when to say, "I used to do that! But wow, I'd need a serious refresher course in order to be proficient in it again!" There's only so much the brain can focus on at once. It's about being honest. With that in mind, let me share some of my self-assessments, starting with hospitals.

Critical care units are full of sounds, smells and sights that many would consider to be horrific. Sensory overload. I got used to it. I think we all got to the point of being able to audibly discern sound frequencies, so we knew for example, when an IV was occluded or empty, even on the regular floors. Sometimes the majority of patients would be so critical, and their care so intense, it would be hard to take a bathroom break. For that reason, I developed a really bad habit of not drinking nearly enough water, or any other fluids for that matter. I hear this can also be the case with many people who are customer service representatives and "on the clock" so to speak. I don't know about now, but I hear it used to be if they had to go to the bathroom, or break for any reason, they were timed. If that is still the case, it's horrible because the needs of the employee have taken a back seat to productivity and profit. I'm aware of the need for businesses to ensure profit, but work conditions on certain jobs come with challenges, let's just say.

There was sympathy, disbelief and frustration, regarding what people did or did not do with and to their bodies. We often wondered how our patients could be so negligent. It was sometimes hard not to be judgmental. Even though we are healthcare professionals, we are still human. Many times, we had to check ourselves, either by sitting quietly and counting blessings; by recalling and having to deal with health or day-to-day issues personally or with our own family members; or through sitting with patients and families talking in as much detail as we had time for, about life experiences.

With some patients, although we tried, the situation was

hopeless. They were broken beyond fixing before they even got to us. Death was a normal occurrence. With others, we celebrated victories. Some illnesses seemed to simply be a test of the resilience of a patient and their family. Some turned out to be a means of forcing needed changes. We couldn't be sure of the whys, but either way, our best practice was consistently necessary.

The regular floors of hospitals were less intense, but frustrating in their own ways. We saw some of the same people return until they could no longer. There was the one with emphysema who still insisted on smoking during his admission. Being able to teach a patient to manage the disease they found themselves with, was our goal so they could live life as normally as possible.

In several home care circumstances, I was older than the patients I was going to see. Whereas many were on 10, 12 medications per day or more, I was on one for a short period of time. I had to lose weight, be more active, pay attention to my body, relax my mind and change my diet. Thank goodness I was able to convince myself to do it. Many people just do not have the energy to do so. For some, life is so full of issues it's not seen as valuable enough to give up certain habits. They would rather have the cigarette or the drinks because that makes them feel better.

Home care was an eye-opener because sometimes it was an adventure. I never knew what I was going to encounter on a first visit. When going to a single-family house, there were times when I wasn't told there was a mean dog, drug activity, etc. Maybe it had been hidden by the family out of fear that they would not be able to get assistance. I remember dogs being removed from the house while I stayed in the car, waiting to be told to come in, and the dog then sitting outside the door looking in the screen at me.

Numerous days, I went home from the critical care units after working the 12-hour shift and sat silently on the end of my bed de-escalating for 20 minutes to a half hour. Hospitals never close. During Cleveland's worse winter weather, because I lived relatively close to the hospital, I would get called and asked to come in when others who lived further away, would be unable to. It was intense for me, as I had two young sons and a husband.

## Falling into Pits

I'm going to digress a bit and go a bit deeper into my own transparency and share with you some aspects and challenges in my life as a young mother, wife, and RN. My nursing experiences have not been without challenges. I have experienced what I call, falling into the pit. I considered whether or not to include this, but transparency is not only a way of keeping things totally legit, it's freeing, and a way to say I am not perfect despite my own attempts at being efficient and effective. This has been a fascinating, sometimes rocky, but ultimately victorious learning experience. It has strengthened me as well as given me even a small level of expertise (if you want to call it that) in a profession that refers to expertise as "practicing" nursing, just like "practicing" medicine.

In addition to what I mentioned in the introduction regarding nursing school, there was the daily walk – the quarter mile in the dark at 5:30 a.m. to catch the bus so I could be on time to clinicals at 7 a.m. There was occasionally having to pick up my toddler in the snow and walk a portion of that quarter of a mile home. Those times were not easy, but they were doable.

There were three pits I had to climb out of. The first one was relatively minor. I was in my second year of nursing school. We were experiencing financial difficulty and I had to take a semester off in order to work. Fortunately, the hospital where I went to nursing school hired student nurses as nursing assistants in our second year of nursing. It was a monetary and experiential blessing. But, having to watch the other students in my class in what had also been my capacity, was very difficult for me. It made me more determined to graduate.

The next semester I was back in school, was able to go through the commencement ceremony with my classmates, and finish up the next semester, taking my state board only five months later. By that time, I had three-week old baby number two. All four of us traveled two and a half hours down the road so I could take the state board because I was breast-feeding. I'd get up, feed him, he'd take a bottle while I was at the testing site all day, and I'd rush back to the hotel to feed him before I burst open. I passed it with flying colors! Good grief, though.

The second pit was a pit of suspension. I was working Neuro/Neurosurgery and wanted to transfer to the SICU. Once I transferred to the SICU, I liked it, but I was very insecure and very intimidated by the scrutiny I felt was coming from the staff. They legitimately wanted not only to get to know me, but to see if I was going to fit into the high-paced, highly technical nature of the unit. It was a friendly environment, but they meant serious business, which was absolutely necessary in a large inner-city teaching hospital. There were all kinds of patients suffering the effects of major accidents, a variety of major surgeries, and other treatments and "stuff," often referred to as train-wrecks.

The problem with insecurity and feeling intimidated was I found it hard to just go ahead and do what I knew needed to be done. I was nervous and afraid, and people sensed my insecurity by the way I acted and responded. Because of this, they'd come into my patient's room to see how things were going. That would make me more nervous and I'd end up so worried about what they were going to think about me, how they'd criticize me or what they'd find that I didn't do, I'd miss the simplest stuff.

During a brief meeting with the head nurse I was calmly told if I didn't come up to speed, I'd be terminated from the unit. After a three-day suspension without pay, I returned. Three days was just enough time for me to think about it, be sad and embarrassed, get angry with myself, then commit to making it work. I knew I could do it and I wanted it badly.

When I returned, I was a different person. Suffice it to say I had no more problems, and when I put in my resignation five years later to begin school nursing, people were sad to see me go. There was another nurse leaving as well, and the word was that the unit was losing family and strength. It was true; that unit was just as much of a family as my blood family. We depended on each other to care for all of the patients, and that included nurses, doctors, therapists, secretaries, housekeeping, pharmacy. Everyone was a part of the SICU. The short of it was, I started off as a weak link in the chain, and that was dangerous. I had to strengthen up or leave, it was that simple.

At any given time in an inner-city school setting, we have students and families who are homeless or otherwise in seriously uncomfortable living situations. Just because some of us work full-time does not make us exempt. The third pit was worse. I don't remember what time of year it was because I blocked it out of my memory, but I was working full-time, 12-hour shifts in critical care. We lived in a modest house we were in the process of buying, but our mortgage had fallen behind. Suffice it to say without going into detail, pointing fingers or having a pity party, our house was in foreclosure. I was tired and had given up. The sheriff's department had contacted us and stated they'd be coming to evict us on a specific date.

Even though I had given up, I still knew the eviction date. Even though I wished it would all go away, my ori kicked in. Even though I was in somewhat of a state of hopelessness, I was still led to call the realtor who had bought our house. I wanted to know if the date could be changed because I had to work. His response to me was, "Ma'am, if I were you, I would call off sick. Otherwise, when you return, your belongings will be out of your house, possibly in the trash or on the lawn, the house will be locked up with new locks and keys, and that will be it." Now let me be clear. I was talking about all of this going on the next day.

As shocked as I was, I had to rise to the occasion for my sons, if for no other reason. It was already difficult enough for them. That night, we were able to secure our new residence, get the keys, and the eviction crew moved us in the next day.

Many will say "God is so good!" or "Look at God!" Let me be crystal clear: yes, He is and to this day, I remain grateful. It was bad but could have been so much worse. But, if my ori had not kicked in, God would have been good in another kind of way, most likely in more dire circumstances possibly including being on the streets for a night, after losing the majority of our belongings. There's a Yoruba proverb that loosely states "God cannot give what one's ori (head) will not accept." I'm always grateful that even with my shortcomings, my ori is still sensible and will come through.

The fourth and final pit was deeper. I was working hemodialysis. It was fascinating and almost as critical as the SICU, but in a different way. I did 10-hour shifts, arriving at a little after 5 a.m. to start at 5:15 a.m. If you know anything about dialysis, you know it's time sensitive in that, you need to start your patients on the machines in a timely manner because the machines need to be prepared for the next patients, who are scheduled back to back. Most patients are on the machine from three and a half to four hours.

The morning of the incident, I arrived on time and pulled the order sheet for the day off the computer. Because dialysis patients have poor to no kidney function, it's important to know "the numbers" to see what medications they would or would not get, as well as the dosages. I do not know if things have changed, but the two common meds I recall back then were Calcijex and Infed. The day started off like any other, but quickly started going sideways. It was a Monday morning and the first thing was a patient who was typically on a Tuesday, Thursday, and Saturday schedule, came in AND needed a blood transfusion. Fine. They delivered the blood, I checked it with another nurse, and went through the process of adding tubing and preparing to hang it. Out of all those times I hung blood in the SICU, not once did I have the lab call and tell me not to hang the blood "if I hadn't already" because they were "not positive" as to whether it had been cross matched properly. I couldn't believe it. Seriously, y'all? Fine. At least they caught it prior to my hanging it.

The day got worse. A patient in his second week of dialysis came to the unit for his scheduled treatment. He was relatively young (fifties), but had a variety of issues, including being blind. According to his wife, he could be very mean, probably because he was angry with his physical condition. The order sheet I pulled off the computer that morning stated the patient needed to receive both the Calcijex and Infed. I gave both in correct dosages at the appropriate times in the treatment. Shortly after giving the Infed, the patient started having an anaphylactic reaction. I opened the chart and flipped through it and found a note stating the patient "might be" allergic to Infed. I was what's called a float nurse, meaning I covered for vacancies. The nurse in the unit regularly had neglected to enter this information into the computer. I immediately called my head nurse and the director of nursing to the unit to show them what was going on. By this time, the reaction had been reversed. Or so we thought.

One hour later, the patient flat-lined and we were unable to revive him. I had to resign that day in lieu of termination, according to state guidelines. The staff was in shock, some were crying, and I was numb. Let me stop right here and talk briefly again, about my spiritual practice. By the time this book is released, I will have 27 years of priesthood in the system of Ifa. Ifa is the traditionalist practice of the Yoruba people of southwest Nigeria, having been to Nigeria three times, Cuba once, and Ghana once. The practice of Ifa is based on Yoruba culture and pre-dates the modern-day practice of Christianity. I grew up in the United Methodist Church, and have recently attended an Afrocentric Catholic and a historic Baptist church in the heart of Cleveland's 'hoods. My spiritual belief, along with the practice and process, is critically important to me. Nonetheless, it can be difficult to always be obedient, especially when the process feels close to impossible to follow, or the timing is bad. This event happened at yet another bad time for me. I was vulnerable, afraid and had not been spiritually compliant, although I was trying to be responsible. I say this because whatever spiritual process you ascribe to, sometimes you may be challenged with needing to do something that's viewed as a leap of faith or even unwise, or it may be something you don't know how to do. Even through difficulties, faith and spiritual process play a huge part in my life and have been priceless in my ability to process the whys and hows. Ifa theology talks about the importance of a good "ori" (head) in life, and how through trials and triumphs, one's ori can make or break us. To paraphrase, the theology also states God and the Heavenly Hosts cannot give what a person's ori will not accept. I was told by my spiritual elders in major Ifa rites of passage and initiation ceremonies, that clinical nursing was not for me. Perhaps it would have been foolish to stop nursing cold turkey since much of the household income came from me. The problem was, I should have been considering what changes I was going to make and implementing a strategy and exit plan, right away. It would have been better than being spiritually shoved into submission! You can either step out on faith, take a leap of faith or wait too long and be pushed.

The benefit to all of this was it got me thinking, and fast. It made me realize that for me, compliance with spiritual practice would be best. I needed to continuously work on me to be the best me. This included mistakes, issues, challenges and all. It also included looking at myself and seeing what I really felt passionate about. The good thing about the practice of Ifa is, the objectives are based on maintaining gentleness of character, personal development and achieving destiny. Without going into detail, let me just say the study and practice has tools and a methodology in place that will allow for the best results in life, if one is amenable to being faithful in their own skin, so to speak. What I mean by that is, Ifa does not take what I call a "cookie-cutter" approach, implying that all things are good for all people. Uniqueness is appreciated, encouraged, and applauded through the sacred liturgy. But like other spiritual journeys, it takes faith, focus and obedience.

I ended up coming out of that situation with a suspension with a stay, meaning I was not restricted from working in any way. A good part of the reason was because of the strong clinical background I had developed through the other two pitfalls, personal and work-related references, and the statement from my director of nursing, who told me she would arrange to get me on at another facility within a couple of days. I politely declined. I knew the deal.

After letting my license lapse for five years due to the trauma of it all, I finally took the required CEU related to stress management, which I ended up teaching for several years at the corporate level for the EAP provider. The real healing came as a result of my letting my license be inactive for those five years. I needed to address myself without the distraction of the very thing I'd been advised not to continue. When I returned to active practice, I went into the school setting and was there until my recent retirement. It was "spiritually acceptable" for a time.

The other weird thing was, the weekend leading up to that fateful Monday, I went through a series of prayers and cleansings in honor of one of my spiritual anniversaries. My biggest prayer had been to remove things from my life that were hindering my overall progress.

Funny, it was the medical director whom I'd never had an actual conversation with; the older white gentleman who'd looked at me side-ways when I started growing my dreadlocks and got my nose pierced at the same time, who gave me the greatest encouragement in a brief, private meeting. He told me to seek personal and spiritual counsel in my own quiet meditation. He said I had to continue to recognize that I was a good nurse, see the goodness in my practice, and know that sometimes things we don't anticipate, happen. He shared a few of his personal experiences related to litigation processes, I thanked him, left the facility, and never returned. He came through for me at a time I never saw coming.

I am clear that this is my very unique reality. I chose a spiritual path that personally and individually advises devotees how to proceed through life. When we seek and get answers, it's best to respond accordingly. There was no further litigation process, the family had their own viewpoint, and they were good with the settlement and final outcome.

I choose to share these stories because traumatic experiences do not avoid people with "good jobs," people who have faith, or people who are trying to do their best. Many families in our communities at large could be doing better but are not for whatever reason. Some of their issues may be what most of us would consider basic, common sense; things any adult should know and do. Either way, the traumatic fallout on our children and other family members can be huge. Even as I write this all these years later, it hurts to imagine my children returning "home" from school while we were at work had I not made that call to the realtor, only to find that their keys did not work in the new locks. They would have climbed up, looked in the windows, and seen no furniture. This was before the time of cell phones, so they'd have had to find a neighbor who was at home and try to call, if they had memorized our work numbers. Then there would have been the stress and embarrassment of the neighbors calling us at work to ask us what happened. Or our sons waiting outside alone, hungry, confused, needing to go to the bathroom and cold. And truth be told, it would have fallen on me because let's just say, that was the reality of the situation and I was exhausted from it.

I think about my incidents when I'm tempted to criticize someone else's family issues too harshly. I have no clue as to what my school children experience when they're not in school. I have no idea what conditions other than disease processes, got some of my seniors or hospital patients into their situations. Trauma is trauma. PTSD (post-traumatic stress disorder) can manifest in many ways, for many reasons, and can take years to resolve.

## Societal Issues

Growing up in my perfectly imperfect world, I did everything on the correct timeline. Graduated from high school "on time" after getting good grades and participating in extra-curricular activities. I had both parents, a brother and sister, and a dog living in the house. We attended church on Sundays. We knew and got along with grandparents, uncles, aunts, cousins, etc. We had friends who were being raised the same way. We were taught trouble-shooting and problem-solving skills. And all three of us were sent to college. It was not perfect, but it was still good.

Please understand the following observations are personal. I've been taught to observe, evaluate and assess, formulate an opinion, and hopefully come up with possible solutions. You may not agree with me. But remember, a 'hood or neighborhood takes on the face of its inhabitants. Additionally, as I move along my life's timeline, some things I saw in home care for example, became things for me to seriously consider. So, let's start there.

Humans are living longer. There's an entire population of aged adults who require services and support. Studies of the phenomena of aging were said to have begun in the 1930s and 1940s, with more focus given in the 1970s. This gave birth to the field of gerontology. Fast forward to my recent practice in school nursing and issues related to pediatrics. When society has obligations to the care of children as well as elders, with both groups needing special attention for their safety and well-being, we end up with what you may already know to be "the sandwich generation." In addition to living their own lives and attending to their own needs, people are finding themselves caring for or helping address the needs of their children, as well as their parents.

Innovative procedures are making it such that babies born with major afflictions are more likely to have those afflictions addressed, prolonging their life potential. Even though they may be wheelchair bound, cannot talk, cannot feed or toilet themselves, and even though we may not know how much information they can process, they're still members of society and they require care and attention. One child I know of was born within normal limits, with no physical or emotional deficits. However, due to a near drowning episode, the child is now non-verbal, immobile, wheelchair bound, unable to feed or toilet himself. Totally dependent due to brain damage.

I've had people ask me why children "like this" are in school; what can they learn? That can vary; we don't always have a measuring gauge to make that determination. Many may not "learn" anything. They may simply benefit from the sensory stimulus they get from being around others. Additionally, their parents, family members and caregivers still must be afforded the opportunity to earn a living and live their lives, even with the challenge of caring for special needs family members.

Then there's the internet. I like my social media and love being able to go on the internet and search for all kinds of useful information, such as descriptions of medications new to the market, carbohydrate counts, facility locations and contact information, online shopping and much more. But in addition to things that are right, there are many things on the internet that are just plain wrong, misconstrued or otherwise twisted due to our mental and emotional health, environment and choices as humans. At any given time, people use social media to destroy others. Like, adolescent and teen girls who have been convinced to take a nude selfie on Facetime or other video or photo media, and the recipient posts it. Not a wise thing to do, and a very hard lesson. You can only imagine what talking to a teenage girl who has been exposed partially nude online, is like. Especially when the post goes anywhere near viral. Even adults who should know and do better, can be stupid, mean-spirited, conniving, crooked, bullying, provoking and to use the youth's term, petty.

Advertisements for top-of-the-line cell phones, the "best" clothes, bling jewelry, fingernail art, hair weaves, purses and shoes, and beauty treatments that cost way more than what's regularly in the bank account if there's an account, are prominently displayed on the internet for all to imagine and long for. But there are high levels of unemployment or underemployment, low salaries and wages, and the issue of being undereducated. Priorities have shifted and all of this does not line up.

Little Debbie is in second grade and has green dye in her pretty naturally blonde hair, but her front teeth are visibly rotting and black in color. Her mouth looks like the stereotypical definition of meth mouth. Lakisha has thick, two-foot long pink and blue extension braids down her back, but she frequently doesn't have her homework and is failing fourth grade. Fifth grade boys are up on school nights until 1 a.m. because their 19-year-old brother is responsible for them at night. They're not sure where mom is and may not know their dad. They come to school to the nurse first thing in the morning because they have a headache and "don't feel good." I guess they don't, especially since they had to get up at 6 a.m. to catch the school bus, did not eat breakfast, and the last night's dinner was questionable.

Then there's the mom came into school declaring out loud in the main office in front of other adults and children she did not know, that she "turned tricks" to have money to buy Christmas gifts for her children. Way too much information to be told to random people in public.

I certainly do not begrudge anyone for wanting nice things and again, I'm not here to pass judgement. But these are not isolated scenarios and if you do not work in the environment, you may not see them. "Nice things" can help boost a person's mood or disposition tremendously. Despondency, hopelessness and depression can be horrible. But material things are bandage fixes that will not last. It's about prioritizing and at least beginning the process of shifting realities, bit by bit.

Given the problems adults face that trickle down to children, we find ourselves sometimes needing to deal with teenagers on an adult level. I do this understanding I have numerous teachable moments where I can provide mature perspectives and options. Questioning students about how they feel about consequences stemming from their behavior oftentimes causes the student to think, even if they don't have an answer. I've had to tell students on any number of occasions, why it's highly disrespectful to swear at and call adults, vulgar names. Or call anyone names, for that matter. I've told teenage girls why it probably is not a good idea to go on certain job interviews with a tomato red wig on, even though they could be qualified, and even if turned down, it could be viewed as discriminatory. Sometimes asking a question as to why a student is behaving a certain way can turn into a lengthy conversation revealing more than I'd asked for, or it can precipitate an angry reaction.

Here in Cleveland, the number of assaults, car-jackings, and thefts has risen at the hands of youth and young adults who have decided to simply take what they want by force. Fraud has increased, and the behaviors of too many of our students, has seriously deteriorated. Some staff members are afraid of the children and or their family members. Some are tired and simply want to retire, so they therefore hold few expectations and impose minimal. Then there are others who figure out how to stand their ground and expect certain behaviors, knowing their efforts will not result in 100 percent success.

In many families, poor employment, low levels of education, and no skill sets can be generational. There are many single-parent households where the parent is working what would be considered a "menial labor" type job that doesn't pay enough, but it's all they qualify for. There are poor, if any, employee "benefits" that would allow for the flexibility needed to raise children, especially as a single parent. They absolutely cannot leave work but once, maybe twice, or risk being fired.

I have spoken to parents on the phone who were in tears because their child was ill, but they could not leave work to come see about them. They were struggling to pay rent and keep food on the table and were afraid of being fired. In addition to being single parents, some are estranged from their family members, or have ugly situations with baby mommas or baby daddies, to the point where there is no cooperation to benefit the child because the simple-minded adults are tripping. I say simple-minded because, if you can't understand that underage children must be a priority in your partner's life, and you go into that relationship anyway, then there's a serious problem. There need to be agreements with all parties involved. Why adults don't understand that, I don't know. Children are little human beings who depend on the adults in their lives to raise them to be productive, respectable, happy adults. For adults to use children as bait, payback and other things that have little to do with the child, is in my opinion ridiculous and damaging.

Additionally, I can't state it enough: all parents or guardians need to have a viable emergency plan in place, but many do not. This could be because there truly is no help, or it could be due to negligence. Sometimes, I'll get fed a line or a bad excuse. I once told a parent I would not wait an hour, then put her sixth-grade son on the bus with what could have been a dislocated shoulder. No, I was not taking her permission over the phone. This was a 12-year old boy who was considered to be a jock, sitting in my dispensary crying. He was in pain because something was not right. I had to tell her to come, find someone or arrange something, because if she didn't, I would call EMS. And no, I could not accompany him to the hospital because I still had diabetic students that needed to be monitored, and I did not have legal jurisdiction to make decisions for her child. Besides, if something was really wrong with that shoulder, or if her son injured it further while remaining at school or on the school bus, she and some attorney would deny giving me verbal permission for him to go on the bus, saying I "should have made her understand the severity of the situation." That would result in she and her attorney finna get paid, to use 'hood jargon, because of my poor decision or negligence. No, sorry, that was not happening. An emergency plan needs to be in place, and if it changes, the school needs to be notified in writing. After this particular verbal exchange, someone came up to the school with their face balled up into a fist within 15 minutes. I was sitting at the front office desk, waiting. The person looked at me, looked at my badge, said nothing, signed the paperwork, and took the student out.

Sometimes, people want to start stuff because they're angry. I can understand being inconvenienced because I have sons and that's what can happen when you have children. I can also understand stressful situations, which is why I shared two of my own biggest messes. But this is exactly why parents need viable contingency/emergency plans. They cannot do it all! I was blessed to have my parents willing and able to help, especially my father who loved to go get his grandsons when they needed him. There are certain things that must be done if parenting is going to be relatively smooth.

## The Rat Race

"Rise with hope on I face, wishing for better for our human race. Rebuke jealousy out the place, strive together, life is not a rat race." The above are lyrics were written in Jamaican patois or dialect, by Jamaican reggae artist JR Blessington & Str8 Fiyah Band, who gave me permission to share them. I've been blessed to sing background vocals for Mr. Blessington. His lyrics are peaceful, thought-provoking, encouraging and clean. This song is entitled "Hope" on his CD "Hope," which is available through major online distributors. I was led to include these lyrics because of the first sentence, "Rise with hope..." but as I thought about it, the part about life not being a rat race, struck home as well. I was listening to a parent talk about how she was so busy, she didn't know what time it was, only guessing when she went outside and noticed how the sun was positioned. I listen to adults talking of how they commute 25, 40, 60 miles or more a day, to get to work, then do it again to get home at night. Some children are in no after school activities at all, while others are in several. Many children do not play outside, let alone play in some dirt. A whole lot of them do not because their caregiver does not have a washer and dryer. They have to add going to the laundromat to their weekly chores.

Some of our children tell us the strangest things they have for dinner, including chips and candy, if they have it at all. On half days at many schools, lunch is still served, for that very reason. Unfortunately, some caregivers are lazy, but many are tired, do not have cooking skills, are low on money, do not have adequate food, appliances don't work, or they are at work and their children are at home watching themselves. Some parents can be seriously caught up in the rat race of survival.

Speaking of phones, even though our school district policy says students' cell phones can't be on during school hours, countless numbers of children have them on anyway. I've seen second graders with iPhones. Students sometimes have their phones out calling parents to come get them before I've had a chance to speak with them or even assess the student. Seriously, who buys this stuff for a child, but will not see that the same child does their homework? And in our district, I have to also ask, who affords them? Sure, they could be pre-owned, but it could be setting up unrealistic expectations.

As far as long commutes, sometimes it's more lucrative to drive a distance in order to make the extra money. But gasoline prices are high. Some people choose or need large vehicles. Many professionals are single parents, but even two-parent households can feel the rat race.

What about cooking? How many cook from scratch versus going to fast food restaurants? Fast food can be tremendously helpful sometimes, but we won't even talk about the cost, the nutritional value and the whole idea of learning to be self-sufficient. Who gets up to prepare breakfast? Who has time? Schools serve breakfast which is OK because at least the children aren't hungry, but it certainly is not the best from a dietary standpoint.

Here's an example where money was not the issue. Mom is an IT professional, her husband a dentist with his own practice. There were two children in different schools. How early do they all get up to prepare and eat breakfast? Are they going to bed early enough? One requires a several mile commute in busy metropolitan traffic, the other catches a school bus. After school events have to be coordinated. Do you leave your children on the corner to catch a bus and drive on off to work in the morning? Do you let them walk to school alone? And what about participation (that's required in some private schools) in parent teacher associations?

Again, no criticism, just observations and questions. The rat race is not my idea of a good time. Unfortunately, the need to, or simply the desire to do more, have more and be more, can have a stressful effect on a lot of people, and that stress can wreak havoc on people mentally and emotionally. Stress is a known factor in many medical challenges. I don't think life was meant to be a rat race.

## Implications of Medical Innovation and Progress

I began to approach this topic in the previous section. It's one I approach with caution. Remember, even though I talk a lot about children, my experiences prior to school nursing included quite a bit of critical care nursing.

There were many treatments I would consider "radical" and unusual (the Domino sugar treatment, for example). Modern medicine has come up with many ways to allow people to prosper and survive in their own way. While this is a wonderful thing, our schools now need more and more registered nurses and support staff. While many people can be taught to manage certain medical needs, there are legal guidelines and differences in practice for RNs, other healthcare practitioners and support staff. Once again, I'm going to re-emphasize, on any given day, we may be managing insulin dependent (type 1) diabetics on children as young as four or five years old; tube feedings; colostomies; urinary straight catheterization; assisting students who have limited to no mobility; who are non-verbal; who are deaf, blind or have severely limited eyesight; who are organ transplant recipients; who do not speak English; who are homeless; who have significant mental and emotional health issues; who've been molested; and the list goes on. "Managing" means using nursing judgement, which we were trained to do.

Many of these children are in great spirits and have adjusted beautifully. There are others who are not and have not. Adjustments have to be made. It's illegal in many instances to insist that a parent send their child across town to a "special needs" school. Inclusion and mainstreaming are making that a thing of the past, or at least a challenge.

For too many students, older or younger, negativity is the norm. For others, there are few positive role models in the family. Stable families in urban, metropolitan school districts, seem to be having more challenges, and from what I've seen on a daily basis, I have concerns that it will become a bigger problem in a few years. Children of other races, cultures and ethnicities, or even those from more financially affluent families and suburban communities, have their own set of challenges. We know this because all we need to do is look at the issue of the majority of mass school shootings. I choose not to discuss reasons behind this because I've not worked in that environment. Suffice it to say, I have concerns for them and their families, too.

It's up to each community and 'hood, to assess their situations and come up with solutions. This is not to say "outsiders" cannot assist. They most definitely can, but they must be aware that cultural differences are real, and solutions oftentimes center around those specific cultural norms and experiences, and how they view society.

The issue of aging is definitely not exempt. As I continue to go through the retirement process, I find it interesting how the older we get, and as our minds can want and need to slow down, some of the processes seem to be intentionally user unfriendly. Many seniors do not use online and automated services very well for any number of reasons. So, on one hand, we're keeping people alive longer, but not always providing platforms for them to comfortably navigate the system? Sure, there is negligence sometimes. I know some seniors in their 70s who do not have services they qualify for and need. Some of them are very eccentric, some of them have started a level of dementia, some have limited resources including transportation and family ties... It's kind of crazy. And no, I do not have the answers except that every service-providing company needs to have a capable human being in customer service. The automated stuff can be horrible for someone who already has "limits." I'm going to stop on that one, too. But, it's something to think about.

# 7 MOVING FORWARD: A PART OF THE CARE PLAN

So, now what? I say a part of the care plan because I definitely do not know all the answers. Nursing school taught us after the assessment (observation, compiling data, pertinent facts, commentaries and other information), to come up with a care plan. As long as we're in the trenches, we cannot give up the battle. We learn to be creative in our approach and in our solutions. Although I cannot fix all of this, I can do my part. With as many capable people as there are in the world, we can all find our place and do what we can. Over the past 30 plus years, I've taken mental notes and thought long and hard about some things. My jobs were not simply paychecks. They were part of my mission and purpose. Here are some of my thoughts moving forward toward healing. Most of them start with us. Part of my mission is that of a town crier.

## How We Look and Sound, and "Status"

No matter our personality, our initial impression in most cases is visual. How we walk, our posture, the expressions we have on our faces, what we're wearing and whether or not it's appropriate for the environment– all of these things are what leave an impression on a first meeting. If the first contact is by phone, it's our tone of voice, whether we're respectful when addressing a person in their status or role (mother, father, husband, wife, son, daughter, etc.), and our introduction of self. This is important if we want to encourage open dialog. Even if we are upset, a lot of times we need to remember we're upset with the situation, not necessarily a particular individual.

Adults who do not pay attention to their appearance are likely to raise questions. As far as children are concerned, before you say they "should be" focused on their schoolwork, or otherwise learning to mind their business, although that may be true, remember they're children and they're learning. Critical thinking skills are developed gradually, and we're role models. If our appearance is too strange, it will most likely take them longer to process.

When it comes to adults, if my first encounter with a parent, guardian, or other family member is over the telephone, I can usually tell by the conversation how the face-to-face meeting will be. Oftentimes they're surprised when they combine my face, voice and the ID badge. Perhaps I'm a breath of fresh air and the parent may be happy to see a face like mine. Maybe they were reminded that many staff members are old enough to be their parent. The bottom line is I'm responsible for the lasting impression I leave, as well as the first impression.

With any adults, I try to always remember that even if I come to them with a complaint, I have not heard their side of the story, if they even know what's going on. Sometimes lightweight humor helps. My pitfalls help me keep it humble.

In traditional societies, it is expected that the youngest give respect to the oldest, even in sibling lineage. Now, I know some people may not deserve accolades or elder status based on behaviors. This is acknowledged in traditional cultures as well. But the point is, in general, there is a hierarchy, and children as well as adults, need to know that there is, and it doesn't stop with teachers and administrators. It includes cafeteria workers, custodians, security– all employed adults in the school environment.

Additionally, adult to adult, we have to always keep in mind what role we're in. Are we the learner? The provider of information? The information collector? Are we seeking or giving help? Who's the perceived expert? Do we respect or even recognize the person's expertise? I honestly do not want to come incorrect to anyone, even though some situations make me angry. I really don't want to burn the bridge I need to go across before I've even gotten to it!

This is one reason I feel it's important, justified, and necessary that qualified people like me, with natural hair, nose studs, hijabs, and who otherwise present with some cultural influence, are important in as many professions as possible. All children need to see people who look like themselves being successful in their line of work. Children benefit from seeing ethnic diversity, and when they do, they are less likely to learn to label others, as long as acceptance is being taught and not discouraged at home. One couple I know supported their son going to school in his kilt, riding a skateboard. That was the coolest! I remember his dad wore one at his and the child's mom's wedding years ago! I'm quite sure of how the child may have been received wearing a kilt at a school where the children were clueless as to the fact that its traditional men's wear in Irish and Scottish culture. This is unfortunate. I wish we could all celebrate our cultural heritage in peace.

As old as the seniors I visited were, many were still surprised when I'd show up at their door with my ID and their paperwork. It was not uncommon for them to say things like, "Well alright, now! We got a sista nurse!" Certainly, there are many good nurses of all races and ethnicities. But, the more I practice, the more I realize just how limited some people's experiences are.

Remember the story about the woman on public transportation when I was right out of nursing school, who assumed I was working in the food service department? I don't know why she stopped talking to me after I told her I was a nurse. I did not raise my voice or put on airs. I guess perhaps in that moment, I became out of her comfort zone. But, did she not realize that I too was on the bus, as in, using public transportation? Not driving an expensive car. I was holding what I thought was a pleasant conversation with her. And while we're talking about food service, did she realize how very important food is in the healing process? Or how important maintenance and housekeeping are to run a hospital or school? We're talking *teamwork*! Perhaps there are some who look down on these workers. Well, how about if all of the custodians, maintenance workers, food service and housekeeping staff were to walk out for a week? *THEN* what?

Finally, as far as what I said about children and how we present ourselves, let's take it a step further. A couple of years ago, I was at a local high school's all class reunion. Although the alumni were all adults, some brought their children along. At one point, I was line dancing. The music was good, it was hot outside, great company, it was a fun time! When I returned to work Monday, a student came up to me and asked if I'd been at the class reunion and if I was line dancing. I told him yes and asked him why he didn't come say hello. He simply smiled and shrugged his shoulders. Now, just what if I was a drinker and I'd had too much to drink, was a dopehead and had been smoking weed and smelled like it, was dressed inappropriately, or had otherwise presented myself in public in a manner not befitting of a role model, school nurse, or was just not respectable, period? Of course, adults can have fun, but for me, it was yet another reminder of how important it is to use discretion and not be turnt all the way up, in public! (Please refer to our trusty 'Hood Glossary if you are foggy on the definition of turnt.)

## Relating

Despite cautioning myself about being opinionated, I still can be. "What were they thinking?" "I wouldn't do that if I were them..." "I'd do it this way instead..." and so on. Over the years, I've had to continuously remind myself that I am not "them," therefore I may or may not do whatever "it" is a certain way if I were in their shoes. This applies to the way someone is living their life, raising their children, how they choose to dress, how they spend or waste money, foods I see going down the conveyor belt in the checkout line, all kinds of things. I also have to remind myself, situations and thought processes can change and humans can be resilient over time. Oftentimes our worse struggles are exactly what we need in order to develop or even recognize strengths we didn't know we had. Sometimes, this means people will move out of unpleasant circumstances, and it could be because someone totally unrelated, helped instead of judged them. It can be challenging to look past the external to get to the core of the problem, but it's necessary. Life can have a way of making sure our humility is in check. Perhaps this is one reason why those of us who work in human service-related jobs, are more effective if we go through some "stuff" or have some of our own experiences.

Children are interesting. They can be innocently, but brutally honest when they feel they're in a safe environment. Once you gain their trust and respect, you can talk to them about anything. That's why background checks and fingerprinting are mandatory for those who work with them, and that's why inappropriate behavior between adults and children is not tolerated. If you want to help effect change and give them perspectives they can carry into adulthood, you must be relatable. For some, based on individual personalities, this can mean meeting them on their level. I once had a child who I guessed through his behavior, came from a racially biased household. I came to this conclusion based on the manner in which the child tried not to relate to me, how he actually looked at me, and the manner in which he answered me, only when he had to. Add to that, this child was a newly diagnosed diabetic and very angry. I had to let him be angry for a minute. It's a healthy and necessary part of the grieving process. But after several days of coming to school late, missing breakfast, and being found hiding in corners in the hallways on the floor crying, we had a serious, "let's keep it 100" conversation. "This is now your reality" I said to him. "I am your ally. If you need anything, come to me because I'm the only nurse in this building and I want to see you happy and feeling well. Get up and come with me because we're going to get you breakfast. I'm going to tell them you need it even though you're late. Remember, I am your ally, but you must allow me to help you. That means, you will work with me, too." We were fine after that and three years later, he's now well-adjusted with his diabetes and other issues, and pretty happy. I could have been wrong in my initial speculation. But whether I was wrong or right, the behavior was there so I was charged with figuring out how I was going to make things work because as the adult, elder and nurse, it was necessary and expected.

Other things that can help with relatability in schools are, being familiar with social media and even having a positive social media presence; being mindful of how you act in the general public and community at large and taking leadership positions or facilitating extracurricular school activities as able. Actions such as these encourage trust, demonstrate a sense of caring and fun, and they can help facilitate change. Adults need to be genuine and our "brand" needs to be positive.

Effective listening is a major skill to have. This means allowing the energy of the speaker to touch you in such a way that you can sense and then confirm their feelings. It means not telling them how they should feel. It could mean asking them to explain why they felt a certain way. It means trying to put yourself in their shoes. It means understanding that everyone's reality is different, some people's drastically. Everyone's mental and emotional wiring is different, some not being as strong as others, some being made "strong" out of situations and necessity. It means accepting that there are differences, even though it makes you uncomfortable. Be that person for just a minute. For me, it meant being the woman who had granulated sugar poured into her open chest, and then coming out of her induced coma to be told such. It meant imagining how it might feel if I were told I'd need insulin injections daily for the rest of my life. Or imagining being homeless with my mom and three siblings, but still coming to school. It could have meant being that kindergartener who had a dead mouse wedged into the toe of the gym shoe she was wearing. Sometimes, it's best to listen and wait a while before talking. The first thing after expressing sympathy or other concern might be to ask a question, "How do you feel? What do you need? What would help?"

Identifying reasons for dysfunction and following up with a game plan is productive. Simply saying "that's just how I am" and then not addressing it like there's no solution, is something else. Granted, sometimes there is "no solution." I've had several one-on-one conversations with older teenagers where the behavior or issue continued because neither the child nor parent had the interest, focus or energy to change. And consider the older gentleman with emphysema who continued to smoke in the hospital despite his diagnosis. No one can be forced to change a behavior unless they really want to.

That leads to the next thing. It's quite alright to help find assistance and not always be the assistance. Sometimes, we're tempted to individually take on too much. Those of us working in service professions would do well to identify as many other support services as we can, and do not be afraid to refer or make an introduction. Biting off more than we can chew serves no one.

Then there's the issue of recognizing and accepting our own truth. Honesty is critical. If we who work in any type of social, family or children's services, know our thought and opinions are narrow; if we know we have low tolerance levels for different life-styles; if we're impatient; if we know we like things a certain way and have challenges when they are not; and if we cannot or do not want to adjust, it's alright. We just need to be honest, admit it and find something else to do.

## Inner Reflections

Let's consider the saying I referred to earlier "wherever you go, there you are." Oftentimes I wonder what I could have done better with my own children. What's my role in society now? What aspects of my personality do I put out to the public daily? Is it benevolent or otherwise? In what areas can I try to improve myself? I find it necessary to regularly sit quietly to reflect, journal and determine where I can make personal adjustments. I also think back to the disastrous events and narrow escapes of my own life. Writing about my "pitfalls" brought out emotions I must have blocked so I could get through the experiences. Revisiting and explaining them on paper brought the embarrassment, frustration and sadness out, all over again. I didn't want to talk to or communicate with anyone while sprawled across my bed, rehashing that unhappy period of time. I especially considered how much worse it could have been for my sons, and how it would have been for some school staff member to deal with them, just like I've dealt with children in crisis. I thought about how irritable and short-tempered some staff members can be with patients, and although not an excuse for rudeness, I wondered what might be going on in their lives. Crises, transitions or other unpleasantries could be going on at any time in people's lives, causing them to be less than cordial. While personal or familial challenges are not justification for poor behavior, they are real and affect us all differently depending on our coping mechanisms.

## Self-Care

In order to support ourselves and sometimes family members, most adults are required to have a job. That means, being in the midst of and cooperating with other people on a regular basis. Some days, we just might not feel like it. We may not like people due to what's going on in our personal lives. We may not feel like talking or being spoken to. If we're in a service profession, we may consider our problems to be bigger and more critical than those of the clients we're working with, and we may not want to listen to what we consider to be whining.

It's important to have escapes and releases– those things that help us get through life. They can be our religious or spiritual beliefs, hobbies, other income-producing activities that allow us to utilize gifts and talents, such as music performance, or other activities we enjoy participating in.

If we are church goers or if we ascribe to any religious belief system or regimen, how is that working for us? Do we apply the doctrines to our every-day lives? Do we study? Are we of service? Do we have a supportive and active faith community? For those who can afford them, nice vacations can provide needed relaxation and change of scenery.

For those who cannot, natural resources in your city, like lakes, rivers, parks, beaches, etc., can be very healing. If you live in a climate that has cold and intense wintery weather, you may not get all the vitamin D you need. A supplement may be recommended by your healthcare professional if you discuss this with them. Never be afraid to ask for assistance with maintaining a positive outlook and a good mood!

With current trends towards health and fitness, one thing I appreciate greatly is the gym. I keep two yearly gym memberships up, at opposite ends of town, even though I cannot always go as much as I'd like. Three or four days a week does not always happen, but I will always make my way back, keeping track of my progress with my gym diary. I also employ the services of a personal trainer from time to time. A personal trainer was one of the best investments I made in myself nine years ago. Only twice a week for two years straight, made a huge impact. The routine made exercise become habit, and with consistency, my body and mind responded well. As difficult as a workout routine can be, it's very satisfying and makes me smile!

Do *not* underestimate the benefits of a good endorphin rush, or the feeling you get after strenuous exercise! Endorphins are described, using an online dictionary definition, as "any of a group of hormones secreted within the brain and nervous system and having a number of physiological functions... causing an analgesic effect. As far as their ability to reduce our perception of pain, and trigger positive feelings in the body, they act similarly to drugs such as morphine and codeine..." I can attest to the fact of feeling really good after a strenuous workout and sweat. Of course, it feels best if you've been maintaining a routine for a minute, as beginning an exercise regimen can take time to get used to, and you can be really sore! But if your doctor or healthcare practitioner has given you the green light for exercise, push through the temporary discomfort and give it a try. Although strenuous exercise is not for everyone, for many it can be very beneficial. And, we know exercise is not limited to the gym. There's yoga, line dancing, tennis, swimming, boxing, riding a bicycle, walking, etc. All kinds of ways to get moving.

With all I've observed and experienced, I do my best to focus on blessings and being in a state of gratitude. I'm extremely grateful to, as far as I know, be healthy and physically fit. One way I demonstrate praise and gratitude is by doing what I'm able to do. I work out because I can, and I'll continue to as long as I'm able. I have a list of women who continue to inspire me, and I let them know I'm grateful for their motivation. My sharing is in hopes of keeping it going.

Finally, journaling can be extremely cathartic, especially if you have a secure place to put it where no one will violate the private nature of it and read what you wrote. During particularly difficult processes over the years, I've learned to journal my thoughts and feelings. The pages of a journal can and will absorb any of the emotions you feel. It's between you, the pages, the ink pen or the pencil. Write what you're thinking and feeling, then periodically go back and read what you wrote so you can assess your progress. If you've made progress, it's a cause for celebration. If you have not, it's a time to re-evaluate and see why. Professional counseling could be needed. Know that there are not "quick fixes." Maintaining emotional health is a process and can take serious effort.

## Study, Continuing Education and Fun

Admittedly, I got weary of being given more and more to do. But times change, and updated new information becomes available. There are some things I have no real interest in or passion for but still need to know. Then there are the things I'm inspired by and have a deep interest in.

The body's response to food, water and exercise is fascinating to me. I study and promote it as it relates to maintaining wellness. I don't "like" diabetes, but I find it interesting because of the need to manage food, water and exercise along with insulin dosing. Managing food, water and exercise can be beneficial to anyone, even without managing insulin.

In 1992 I started West African dance training and have taken numerous dance classes, workshops and master classes, and have performed at numerous venues, mostly small, but some pretty significant. The learning process included other dance forms like modern, belly and liturgical dance forms. As a result, since I like to encourage fitness in both children and adults, I've taken dance into schools, churches, hospitals and neighborhood organizations. This includes beginner's choreography for adults and children with different needs and abilities.

I am not a professional dancer, but I'm experienced in it and have studied the body through nursing. We do not have to be professionals in all things we choose to share outside of our chosen occupation, as long as we know what we're doing, are good at it, and do not promote injury. I select dances I know and can teach well, and incorporate muscle movement, stretching, rhythm and cardio awareness. Sharing a little bit can go a long way, and it's fun!

## Choosing Our Part in the Solution

If you didn't know before, you now know a small bit of what nurses do. As much as I liked nursing and found it rewarding, it was not the whole of me. What is your profession, and what is the rest of you? What are you passionate about? What annoys you to no end that you need to avoid? Don't be afraid to make adjustments. Some people even change careers altogether. You just need to have a plan and an exit strategy.

A proverb from sacred Ifa liturgy says "How do we eat the head of a rat? It is bit by bit we eat the head of the rat." In other words, a slow, methodical process. And, I know. Rat. Ugghh. It's a type of dried bushmeat (rodent) they eat in West Africa. Think of it as being like that specialized dried jerky stuff, they can charge a lot per pound for here in the United States. My spiritual family over there never offered it to me, thank goodness.

Life consists of a series of choices. We have free will. We can choose to participate in keeping things the same or facilitating change. What'll it be? It's in our hands.

In the meantime, here's to nursing; I loved you! And here's to the 'hood; I love you, too!

# END WITH GRATITUDE

Thank you to all of my patients, students and clients, young and old, who shared their lives with me willingly or unwillingly, whether they were expecting to or not, under victorious or tragic circumstances. I admire your strength and tenacity. I pray I was as much of a blessing to you as you were to me. May the legacies of your fights and struggles as well as your victories, live on anonymously through these pages. May your stories help with healing others. You have added richly to my life and I greatly appreciate you.

 - #Nurse Barbara

# ABOUT THE AUTHOR

Barbara J Barrett, B.Ed, RN also known as Nurse Barbara or BBBeyondCategory, has been taking every 15-minute vital signs, changing dressings, shaking her head at older folks, making jokes in stress management lectures, sitting quietly through Critical Incident sessions, explaining EAP services, counting carbs, calculating insulin dosages, giving tube-feedings, laughing at kids being kids and otherwise navigating her way through a 30-plus year career as a registered nurse. She has a huge appreciation for nursing because the other side of her is the artist at heart, who benefits from the mental grounding required to be a proficient nurse. When she's not nursing you can hear her singing lead vocals live with her own band, lead or background with other bands, or in the recording studio. Genres range from classic jazz, neo-soul and reggae, to European classical, gospel, R & B and blues. You may see her on a local or national television commercial; dancing primarily West African or liturgical dance; see her in small acting roles onstage or see costumes she's created for actors on various stages in the local world of community theater. She's a student/initiate in the traditionalist practice of Ifa, a spiritual counselor of many, a mother, a "GMa" and a lover of life. Check out more at: www.bbbeyondcategory.com and of course www.hoodmedical.com You can also visit on Facebook, Instagram, LinkedIn, and YouTube

*#bbbeyondcategory #nursebarbara*
*#nursevocalist #hoodmedical #thisiswhyising*